Root of Thought

✦

Reflections on Neuroscience

Henry Kong M.D.

iUniverse, Inc.
New York Bloomington

Root of Thought
Reflections on Neuroscience

iUniverse books may be ordered through booksellers or by contacting:

iUniverse
1663 Liberty Drive
Bloomington, IN 47403
www.iuniverse.com
1-800-Authors (1-800-288-4677)

Because of the dynamic nature of the Internet, any Web addresses or links contained in this book may have changed since publication and may no longer be valid. The views expressed in this work are solely those of the author and do not necessarily reflect the views of the publisher, and the publisher hereby disclaims any responsibility for them.

ISBN: 978-1-4502-2267-9 (pbk)
ISBN: 978-1-4502-2269-3 (cloth)
ISBN: 978-1-4502-2268-6 (ebook)

Printed in the United States of America

iUniverse rev. date: 5/6/10

Dedicated to the Parents:
Wonsil Kim Kong
Young Duk Kong
Anne Treisman
Michel Treisman
Danny Kahneman

& the Teachers:
Francis Crick
Richard Dawkins
Dan Dennett
Steven Pinker
Vilayanur Ramachandran

In appreciation of the two most brilliant cultures of all time:
The English and the Jews, and my brilliantly cultured English Jew, Jessica Treisman, for the proofreading, back cover photo, and much else.

Special thanks to Josh Sanes, Jean Livet, and Tamily Weissman for the beautiful cover photo of mouse hippocampal neurons labeled with the 'brainbow' system.

Thanks to Jonah Lehrer and Michel Treisman for the positive comments.

Contents

Foreword

Henry Kong, the author of *More Self than Self: At Autism's Edge* and the three-volume *History of the Universe,* has set his talents to an even more challenging task. In this book, his focus is on the neuronal and genetic underpinnings of the thought patterns that make us uniquely human: consciousness, judgment, religion and politics. In a conversational style that makes even the details of neuronal circuitry easy to follow, Dr. Kong takes the reader through the latest findings of developmental biologists, neurophysiologists, cognitive and social psychologists, and evolutionary biologists. Did you know that conscious thought and perception account for only a very small proportion of your mental life? Have you ever wondered why thinking through the alternatives sometimes just makes it harder to make a decision? Did you know that seizures in a particular part of the brain can induce deep spiritual experiences? Would you be surprised to learn that you were born with specific political preferences? Root of Thought digs deep into the brain to answer these questions and many more. The book is a thought-provoking exploration of how our mental lives have been shaped by biology over the course of evolution.

Jessica Treisman
Professor of Molecular Genetics
Skirball Institute
NYU School of Medicine

Introduction

The prominent neuroscientist and public intellectual Vilayanur Ramachandran has called the human mind the greatest mystery in the universe. Fascinating and complex, certainly, but I don't think it needs to be so mysterious. Over the last two decades, the three hitherto unrelated fields of cognitive neuroscience, developmental genetics, and evolutionary psychology have converged to answer some age-old questions about how and why three pounds of fatty tissue gives rise to the totality of our mental lives. Our understanding of the modular architecture of the brain, the genetic basis of neural development, and the evolution of cognition have grown exponentially in the process. We are now living in the midst of a truly golden age of exploration on par with that of Captain Cook and Isaac Newton. The purpose of this book is to share some of the strange and wondrous discoveries of neuroscience with the curious lay reader.

I am a physician in private practice in a largely geriatric community in central New Jersey. I recently took care of a pleasant lady in her late eighties. Aside from some early signs of dementia, Florence was living independently and doing relatively well. Then one morning she presented to my office complaining of fatigue and headaches. A routine blood test revealed an elevated platelet count, which, though not specific, may herald the onset of cancer. I hoped she would improve on her own, but on a follow up visit, her symptoms persisted, and her abnormal platelet count was even higher. I referred her to a hematologist who ordered a special blood test to look for a genetic mutation called *bcr-abl* that causes blood cells to multiply out of control. She had this mutation, which meant that her diagnosis was *chronic myelogenous leukemia*, a cancer of the white blood cells. She was hospitalized and treated with a special drug that targets and kills mutant cells. Unfortunately, it was too late. Florence was producing abnormal blood cells faster than we could remove them. They clogged up the blood vessels in her heart and brain, causing her to have a heart attack and a stroke. Her immune system became too weak to fight off bacteria, and her bloodstream became infected with an antibiotic-resistant staphylococcus. Realizing the inevitable, her family agreed to have her transferred to hospice care, where she was kept comfortable with frequent cocktails of morphine and tranquilizers. Her mind deteriorated from her baseline mild dementia to delirium to unconsciousness before her body finally shut down.

Florence's case made me think about consciousness and the identity of the individual. Throughout her illness, her family kept their spirits up and requested all reasonable treatments for her cancer and its complications. Never mind that her blood was filled with genetic mutants that crowded out her healthy cells, never mind that her cognition had declined from Alzheimer disease, never mind that foreign bacteria had infiltrated her body, there was still something about Florence that made her Florence, and that was enough to give her family hope. But once she slipped into coma, they conceded that she was no longer 'there', and accepted her inevitable demise. Florence's case illustrates the natural human tendency to define a *self* as the function of a conscious mind. As long as a person reports that she experiences and remembers the world from a certain point of view, we recognize her as a self that is integrated over space and time, regardless of what may happen to her physical body. But if she loses the ability to experience and remember, we say that she is no longer herself.

The central question of consciousness is the topic of my first chapter. Without going into detail here, let me say that consciousness is simply an evolutionary adaptation, just like a lion's claws, a butterfly's wing patterns, or the flocking behavior of birds. It evolved in our ancestors because it was useful for social life, just as claws were useful for catching prey, or colorful wings were useful as sexual displays, or flocking was useful for safety. Some might argue that consciousness is too complex to be a mere adaptation. But the roots of complex thought are there to serve a purpose.

Three main stumbling blocks have hindered our scientific understanding of consciousness. First, consciousness is the only tool we have to understand anything, including consciousness itself. We can describe pointy claws and flocks of seagulls using other measuring sticks, but with consciousness, it's like lifting yourself up by your own proverbial bootstraps. Second, no other animal has a language to describe its conscious experience. This makes it rather difficult to partake in comparative studies of consciousness. Third, consciousness is wrapped up in a huge range of complex behaviors from technology to mythology to culture and custom. The tree of the human mind is big and gnarly, with lots of tangled branches and thick foliage. But I believe that by applying the powerful reductionistic approaches of computational neuroscience, gene science, and evolutionary theory, we can dig down to the very roots of thought.

A hundred thousand years ago, all of our ancestors were Africans. The entire human race numbered no more than a few thousand individuals confined to a precarious existence in the arid landscape of the Great Rift Valley. These ancestors may have resembled modern day Bushmen of the Kalahari, and perhaps spoke a click language similar to theirs as well. African Adam and Eve mark the root of human culture, but not the root of thought. To get there, we need to go much further back. It is likely that some form of consciousness had been well established in East Africa for several million years. The great apes evolved from monkeys who already possessed most of the neural circuits (and the genes for building them) necessary for the types of cellular computation involved in language and social decision-making. We now know that rhesus macaques have special cells called *mirror neurons* that fire not just when the creature does something, but also when it sees someone else doing the same thing. It is just a short step to adapt a mirror system useful for predicting another's behavior to a full-fledged mindreading system designed for understanding another's thoughts. Professor Ramachandran has speculated that the mindreading system may then have been turned upon itself to reflect the thinker's own thoughts. Thoughts about one's own thoughts: isn't that what self consciousness is?

Consciousness is a clever adaptation for life as a social ape. But like all adaptations, it has its limits. Lion claws and butterfly wings are made of tissue and proteins that require proper diet and maintenance to keep their integrity. Likewise, a fully functioning conscious system is a phenomenon that requires a well-nourished neural substrate to keep it going. It is important to point out that a healthy brain is necessary but not sufficient for consciousness, because not all that is brain is conscious. There are great swaths of brain that are crucially important for maintaining the vegetative functions of homeostasis such as breathing, heartbeat, temperature, and sleep. And just as Freud correctly anticipated, there are neural organs that subserve reflexes, facial expressions, and even full-fledged perceptions, memories, and behaviors that do not enter the realm of conscious thought at all. In fact, the landscape of the human mind is mostly under the surface of consciousness. Consciousness is a recently evolved anomaly that takes up only a small part of our mental activity. But ironically, this adaptation exaggerates its own potency, falsely convincing itself of its suzerainty over the rest of the mind. It is this selfish delusion that makes it so difficult for the mind to understand itself.

In the later chapters, I will shine a light on decision-making, religion, and politics from the dual standpoint of the subconscious mind and its conscious interpretation. It is from the uneasy tug-of-war between these two entities that the weirdness of behavioral economics, magical thinking, and moral philosophy arise. Public policy, national interests, and, increasingly, even the fate of the human species hinge on how we deal with the technological and environmental implications of our collective decisions. Ultimately, it is the conscious mind that makes the final judgment. But it is profoundly influenced by the rest of the subconscious brain. It would serve us well to learn as much as we can about the different parts of the mental world and how they work together.

Chapter 1

Consciousness

'You', your joys and your sorrows, your memories and your ambitions, your sense of personal identity and free will, are in fact no more than the behavior of a vast assembly of nerve cells and their associated molecules.

Francis Crick
The Astonishing Hypothesis

Stephen Colbert: In five words or less, how does the brain work?
Steven Pinker: Nerve cells fire in patterns.

The Colbert Report

How does it feel?

Close your eyes. Clear your thoughts. What comes to mind? The fading orange of the setting sun, perhaps, or the window frame, or your fingers holding the pages of this book. Try as you might, these pictures cannot be separated from one another in space and time. The details fill in and melt together effortlessly. Your attention captures a vivid here and know that just as quickly slips away.

The image in your mind's eye is neither frozen nor flat; it is a space with depth, length, and height. Colorful shimmering impressions move in and out of focus. The leaves of a sycamore tree rustle in the evening breeze. Its shadow lengthens towards the cornfield and the farmhouse beyond. It's getting harder to make out the details in the gloaming, but you know they're out there.

Sit up, walk to the window, unlock the hinge, and lift. It's stuck. Pull harder; more tugs until it suddenly gives. Slide it up past peeling paint chips. Now step back, close your eyes, and concentrate again. What fills your senses? The sound of birdcalls, the smell of freshly-mowed grass, the heat on your fingers all share space in your mind's eye, but not all at once. Now open your eyes. You may recall reading a book like this once before, when you were in college. But the scent of a late summer evening suddenly brings forth memories from many years ago. Was that you?

*****

All organisms have been naturally selected over millions of generations to survive and reproduce in their own particular niche. In the case of animals, evolution has invented sensory systems that enable monitoring of the external world in real time and motor systems that allow self-propulsion. The behavior of these input/output systems is largely hardwired, either at birth or shortly thereafter, through the elaborate unfolding of genetic programs. Every organism has an identical set of genes (about 23,000 in the case of humans, and 18,000 in the fruit fly) in each of its cells. This genetic ensemble contains the recipe for sculpting the entire creature. But not all genes are expressed at the same time or in the same cell. Gene expression is regulated by complex interplay of the environment with other genes, which themselves are usually controlled by yet other genes, such that their protein products are made at specific sites and times in the animal's body and lifespan. The result is the differentiation and development of specialized cells such as liver cells, blood cells, and muscle cells, and the organization and growth of those cells into specialized tissues and organs such as skin, heart, and brain.

At the genetic level, lower animals such as nematode worms and fruit flies are nearly as complex as human beings. The number of genes they possess and the way they are regulated are not very different from us. In fact, thanks to the conservative nature of evolution by natural selection, most human genes have counterparts in insects and worms. This makes them ideal model organisms for scientific and medical research into things like cancer, heart disease, and diabetes. Having evolved from a common ancestor hundreds of millions of years ago, humans and all the 'lower creatures' on earth truly are cousins.

At the level of the brain and mind, however, things begin to diverge. Insects and worms have neurons quite similar to ours. But because of their small size, their brains are necessarily less complex. As a result, their behaviors are rather stereotypical. Whether these creatures of habit have minds is difficult to answer (I would guess no), but we can be fairly certain that if they do, they would be markedly impoverished compared to ours.

As we proceed to the higher organisms (vertebrates, mammals, monkeys, and apes), there is a trend towards greater neurological complexity. All complex biological behavior is the product of brain activity, via the neuromuscular interface. Increasing neural complexity is almost always accompanied by increasing behavioral complexity. Higher animals do not necessarily act predictably. Their behavior is flexible and adaptable to the environment. They learn. And one species of primate in particular, Homo sapiens, has learned to reflect upon its own behavior. This ability is made possible by a generous grant from the human cerebral cortex.

Perception

Behavioral flexibility depends on the proper functioning of many parts of the brain. At the very beginning of this process is sensory perception. Organisms act in response to what they take to be 'out there'. Neuroscientists now have a rather good picture of at least the first stages of perception. We know that touch, balance, hearing, smell, sight, and taste are mediated by minute receptors in the skin and joints, in structures deep inside the ear and nose, in the retina at the back of the eye, and in taste buds on the surface of the tongue. These receptors translate or transduce phenomena in the outside world like heat, gravitational acceleration, odor molecules, and waves of sound and light into patterns of electrical activity on the surface membrane of sensory nerves. Perception occurs as the information conveyed by these patterns is relayed to higher and higher processing centers in the central nervous system.

Let's take the often-used example of vision. Imagine light coming from the outside world passing through a lens and focused into a tiny upside-down image on a thin curved sheet of retinal nerve cells in the back of the eye. There, specialized receptor cells, the rods and cones, contain chemicals that change shape when energized by absorbing light. These chemical reactions produce changes in the electrical potential of these cells that are transmitted to neurons connected to them. If sufficiently stimulated, these neurons will produce electric spikes, or action potentials, which spread down their axons and are passed on to other neurons that may be linked to them. They are, in effect, tiny electrical wires made of organic molecules rather than copper. The activities of thousands of nerve cells are channeled into multiple bundles of neural code streaming from the two eyes through the arching optic nerves. These nerves cross the optic chiasm, pass through a relay station known as the lateral geniculate nucleus of the thalamus, and arrive at an area at the back of the brain called V1, the primary visual cortex. The perceived visual image that was initially projected onto a thin sheet of cells on the surface of the retina is transferred to another thin sheet of cells at the back of the brain. But that image is no longer made of light, but by a representational digital code contained in millions of neurons. Objects to the right side of your nose (your right visual field) stimulate the left side of the retina on both eyes and eventually end up on your left visual cortex. Objects on the left side end up on the right visual cortex. This cross-over phenomenon, known as decussation, is a curiously common motif found throughout the nervous systems of all higher organisms. Other sensory modalities such as touch, pain, and hearing (but not smell), as well as the control of motion of one side of the body are also processed in the opposite side of the brain.

The picture we see out there now exists in the form of a partially processed buzz of electrochemical activity spread out over millions of nerve cells and their billions of connections, called synapses, scintillating with the bursts of millions of action potentials. Believe it or not, there is order in all this noise. Back in the 1960's, the great pioneers of modern neuroscience, David Hubel and Torsten Wiesel, discovered that patterns of neural activity in cats and monkeys actually code for simple features like edges, movements, and colors in particular parts of the visual field. Each neuron in the visual pathway has a receptive field, a region of space within which a stimulus will produce a response in the neuron. Retinal cell receptive fields are sensitive simply to spots of contrasting light, for example, a dark spot surrounded by light, or a light spot surrounded by darkness. A single cortical cell receives information from several retinal cells and summates the information from their simple fields. As a result, cortical receptive fields are more elaborate; they depict lines and edges rather than spots. Cortical neurons still further up the line then summate the information from the lower level cortical cells, producing even more complex receptive fields. Some of these cells respond to motion, orientation, and shape. Information is organized through the hierarchical architecture of neural connectivity.

The visual field is mapped point by point onto the surface of the visual cortex. Columns of cells in the visual cortex are dedicated to analyzing different features of visual stimuli such as which eye is seeing them, what their colors are, and how their edges are oriented. Neuroscientists have now mapped the primary visual cortex of animals such as cats and monkeys, and it is possible to visualize in stunning full color the activity of the cortical columns in living animals by a technique called optical imaging.

This neural activity is still at the early stages of visual processing. More interesting stuff happens further upstream. The axons of the V1 neurons are intimately connected to many neurons in other cortical and subcortical (evolutionarily more ancient neuron clusters beneath the cerebral cortex) areas. In the 1970's, the neuroscientists Leslie Ungerleider and Mortimer Mishkin observed that the higher order processing of visual input is roughly divided into two pathways: a dorsal stream (so called because its nerve fibers run along the top, or dorsal, part of the brain), and a ventral stream (whose fibers run along the lower, or ventral, part of the brain). The dorsal stream specializes in the location of objects in space, allowing one to perform such tasks as grasping a moving branch or catching a passed football, while the ventral stream deals preferentially with the recognition of objects. Thus the dorsal system has come to be known as the 'where' or 'how to' pathway, and the ventral system as the 'what' pathway. Though somewhat underappreciated at the time, Ungerleider and Mishkin's discovery has turned out to be one of the landmark advances in modern neuroscience with implications extending far beyond perceptual psychology.

There is now much evidence supporting this elegant division of visual perception. Perhaps most impressive are the psychological double dissociation cases of brain injury patients who have deficits in either the processing of motion (such as perceiving the flow of water) or in the perception of form (such as recognizing simple geometric shapes), but not both. These patients were subsequently found to have anatomic lesions in either the dorsal or ventral systems, respectively.

The other sensory systems are designed similarly. Sounds, touch, temperature, tastes, and smells are all deconstructed and then recreated in their respective areas of the brain. A different area of cortex is allocated for each modality. This deconstruction is followed by integration in association areas of the cortex where combinations of features are bound together to create a fairly accurate facsimile of the outside world. How does an object maintain its apparent integrity even though its features take separate routes through the perceptual system? This question has come to be known as the binding problem. It is one of the great unsolved questions in neuroscience today. There are actually three separate binding problems. More on this later.

The products of our perceptions are not, of course, the real world; they are working approximations of external reality. A typical theater stage set consists of numerous cheap props. Taken alone and offstage, they look artificial. But taken together and under proper lighting, they imbue a scene with meaning and believability. So it is with the mind's eye. We do not see a circle of blackness where our natural blind spot (the part of the visual field where the optic nerve leaves the retina) is. We are prone to visual illusions that trick us into thinking an object is darker when seen against a light background than if it were set against a darker one. The moon looks much larger on the horizon than it does high up in the sky. This is because our senses have evolved shortcuts to get the job done. Where there is a lack of information, such as the blind spot, the brain simply 'fills in' the gap. Our minds abhor a vacuum; as far as they're concerned, absence of information does not equal information of absence. When accurate perception would require a great deal of computation, such as figuring out the absolute brightness or the actual size of an object, or the stuff that's hidden behind the blind spot, the brain simply makes its best guess. This is a recurring theme that we shall see in various guises throughout this book: the mind is a grab bag of tricks designed by natural selection to get our genes into the next generation. It is created by a process that has no goals or foresight. In the words of the legendary biologist and neuroscientist, Francis Crick, 'God is a hacker.'

Perceptual coherence is an area of intense and exciting research for neuroscientists. An object in the world, such as a wedge of Swiss cheese, activates different sensory neurons specializing in perceiving the sizes and patterns of the holes in the cheese, the smell of the cheese, the color of the cheese, and so on. These cells are activated simultaneously and pass on information to downstream neurons in the association cortex. The simultaneous activity arriving at the association areas acts to bind these disparate properties of the cheese together, thus integrating the perception into a coherent interpretation.

This approximate picture we see in our mind's eye is a remarkably veridical one. The sights and sounds we see and hear seem to emanate from things out there rather than from phenomena in our heads. The explanation is that evolution has made our mental approximations of external reality match very tightly to the physical world, at least in those dimensions that are important for our survival. The view directly down from my girlfriend's 15th floor window above the East Village really does appear to be approximately 150 feet above the East Village. If it did not, perhaps due to a genetic glitch affecting the development of my brain's perceptual circuits, I might be prone to step out into the abyss, forfeiting my chance of passing on any possible altitude misperception genes to my progeny. On the other hand, equally 'real' phenomena like ultraviolet light, magnetic field intensity, relativistic time dilation, or the simultaneous visual perception of all six sides of a cube are inaccessible to our naked senses. This is because evolution has neither felt the pressure to select nor had the biological substrate with which to create the means for sensing them in our species.

Our perception of a coherent reality is a product of complex and creative neural ensembles that simultaneously deconstruct and integrate sensory input. Neurological deficits can interrupt this process. Damage to sensory receptors at the bottom of the pathway causes primary defects such as congenital red-green colorblindness or conductive hearing loss. Damage to later stages of sensory conduction is responsible for cortical blindness or sensory neural hearing loss. Damage to even more upstream areas in the association cortex can result in more specialized deficits. Examples include the previously mentioned inability to perceive motion (optic ataxia) due to lesions in the dorsal visual stream, the inability to perceive shape (apperceptive agnosia) from lesions to the ventral visual stream, and even the inability to perceive faces (prosopagnosia) from damage to the face processing area of the fusiform gyrus.

Why Me?

My earliest memory of self-awareness was as a six-year-old in Mrs. Dixon's first grade class. We were sitting on the school bus on our way back from a school trip to Manhattan. The other kids were jumping around and being rowdy. I remember wondering what caused them to make so much noise. Eventually the proctor stood up and hollered, "Everyone hush up or we aren't leaving!" Most of the kids kept on yelling. A few started to look around with wide eyes and frenzied head turning saying, "Sssssshhhhhh!!!" Then one of them yelled, "Shut up, you guys, shut up, or we don't go home!" I remember thinking to myself that if everyone kept quiet for themselves, then others wouldn't have to make more noise telling everyone else to be quiet. Then I wondered why, if I could be quiet by myself, everyone else couldn't be like me? What was going on in their heads to make them behave in the particular way that they did? This made me imagine all sorts of things. What would it be like to enter someone else's mind? What would it be like to enter my own mind at some point in the past? Do I remain the same person as I get older? Do sensations feel different for different people, or for the same person at different times? These thoughts eventually led to one urgent question for which I have yet to find a satisfactory answer: *of all the people I could have been, why am I... me?* This weird thought grew on me as the bus finally grew quiet and crossed the Hudson that evening.

I remember quite vividly the experience of seeing the rapidly passing cables of the George Washington Bridge pass the slower moving amber tinted clouds of sunset. First, I focused on the cables, keeping them steady as I saw the cars and clouds pass by. Then I focused on clouds, as I saw the cables pass across. My attention shifted from the cables to the clouds, back to cables, back to clouds as the bus sped across the bridge towards the Palisade Cliffs. Then the questions came back, more urgently than before. I AM ME! I am sure of that, but why me? Will I always be me? How did I come to be the center of my universe? The feeling made me feel dizzy with confusion. I sensed I had stumbled on something profound.

*****

Throughout this book, I will describe what the brain does and what causes it to happen. The goal of our journey in this chapter is the mysterious point where all these disparate elements of mind come together and connect to mean something for each of us: consciousness.

Consciousness is at once very easy to understand, yet fiendishly difficult to explain. It is the thread that binds our perceptions and actions into a coherent self. It is also something about which science has had remarkably little to say, until now. Once the purview of philosophers and religious mystics, consciousness is quickly becoming a legitimate target for neuroscientists, computer engineers, and cognitive psychologists. Thanks to them, we are steadily gaining a coherent picture of how the brain creates mind.

The Varieties of Conscious Experience

Before I explain how consciousness happens, I need to define a few loose terms. According to the Oxford American Dictionary: [con-scious-ness n. **1** the state of being awake and aware of one's surroundings and identity (lost consciousness during the fight). **2** awareness; perception (had no consciousness of being ridiculed). **3** the totality of a person's thoughts and feelings, or of a class of these (moral consciousness).] When people commonly speak of 'consciousness' they may be referring to one of at least three types of consciousness. The first type is the subjective feeling or awareness of something. It is what it *feels like for you* to savor a shrimp taco, behold a red rose, suffer a paper cut, have your heart broken, or experience an orgasm. Such feelings can be triggered by an actual object or event in the outside world, a memory, or even a figment of the imagination. These personal feelings are private by definition, and cannot be shared with anyone else. Psychologists have concocted many terms for this aspect of conscious experience including *qualia*, *core consciousness*, and *phenomenal consciousness* (*P consciousness* for short). I will use these terms interchangeably to refer to the same thing.

A second type of consciousness refers to experiences that we can share with others through verbal report. "That shrimp taco at Mercadito was exquisite," "I'll have to remind myself to buy her a dozen red roses for our anniversary," or "that poison ivy episode last summer ruined my vacation" are statements that reflect feelings, memories, and plans translated into language. The translation makes our private thoughts – P consciousness – more overtly accessible both to ourselves and to others. I will call this '*A consciousness*', where A refers to access.

Finally, there is the awareness of oneself as a unitary being or agent experiencing the taste of shrimp tacos, thinking about a dozen red roses, or remembering one's first sexual encounter. This is the experience we have of ourselves as the first person subjective, a fixed point of reference to which all memories, emotions, and perceptions occur. It is the source of all of our decisions, beliefs, and actions. This is the '*I*' who endures through time and travels through space, constantly changing in size, appearance, and health, but remaining the same entity that possesses both P and A consciousness. This is self-consciousness ('*S consciousness*').

I propose that the three varieties of consciousness are actually distinct entities mediated by different areas of the brain. Moreover, in certain pathological cases such as autism or schizophrenia, they are dissociable. Because the mind is what the brain does, we need to examine closely those parts of the brain responsible for consciousness. This is what neuroscientists call the neural correlates of consciousness or *NCC*. But before zooming in on the neurophysiology, I will give you an overall schematic of how the mind constructs consciousness.

A useful way to understand how consciousness works is to take one aspect such as vision or hearing and examine the process from the business end (the eye or ear) to the corporate office (visual or auditory awareness). I will utilize this approach by taking a real life example of sensory input and constructing a model of P consciousness that is applicable to all aspects of sentient awareness including perception, memory, emotion, and imagination.

Kingdom Come
Cambridge, Massachusetts, summer 1988. I was sweating in my Next House dorm room on Memorial Drive looking out at the Boston University campus across the Charles River. Needing to take a break from my med school entrance exams prep book, I took out a new CD I had just bought in Central Square: the heavy metal rock band, Kingdom Come. On track # 9 was the song 'Loving You'. The opening guitar chords resonated in my mind. There was something about it that reminded me of a beach in Southern California. I skipped the CD back to the beginning and listened again and again to the opening riff. The feeling evolved into a vivid visual illusion. I pictured myself walking along a boardwalk gazing out at the ocean. The morning was oppressively hot and the horizon was blurred in hazy chiaroscuro. The chords sounded distant and distorted, as if I were listening to a weak radio signal. I pictured myself languidly walking along that sandy landscape of the mind. What was going on?

Let's analyze this from bottom to top. First, the train of sound waves from the CD speakers stimulates my eardrums. This causes the three tiny bones of the middle ear to move and create minuscule vibrations in the fluid inside the snail-like coils of the inner ear called the *cochlea*. The vibrations stimulate hair like projections on the specialized nerve cells lining the inner ear called *hair cells*. The hair cells are arranged along the length of the cochlea; those at one end have 'long hair' and are stimulated best by low frequency sounds. Those at the other end have 'short hair' and respond best to high frequency sounds. The inverse relationship between length and frequency is a physical principle that explains, among other things, the changing pitch of musical instruments.

The mechanical stimulation of the hair cells causes a biochemical reaction that opens tiny pores on the nerve cell membrane. This allows positively charged calcium and potassium ions to enter the cell. The influx of these ions changes the electrical charge along the axons of the hair cells, depolarizing them. Thousands of stimulated neurons responding to a certain sound send their action potentials through the auditory nerve at fifty meters per second. From there, the signal passes through the brain stem on the way first to the *medial geniculate nucleus* of the thalamus, and then to the primary auditory cortex of the brain. Like the visual system with its retinotopic organization, the auditory processing surface of the thalamus and the cerebral cortex are arranged in a precise spatial order. The neurons representing high frequency sounds are located towards the front and those representing low frequency sounds are located in the rear of both the thalamus and the auditory cortex. This is called *tonotopic representation*.

Surrounding the primary auditory areas in the temporal lobes are the supplementary and higher order auditory association areas of the brain. These areas possess their own separate, more complex tonotopic maps. The sounds of the guitar chords are represented and processed here. From the ear to the auditory cortex, sound waves are transduced into electrochemical signals and bundles of action potential spikes whose patterns are represented in auditory maps on the surface of the brain. But none of these 'musical pictures' are in consciousness…yet. The same is true for all the other sensory modalities: vision, taste, smell, touch, pain. To become conscious of these things, we need to go even further up (Figure 1).

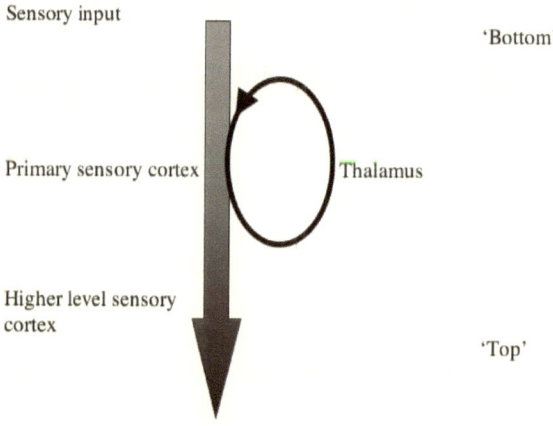

Figure 1: Perception

Sensation

The neural codes representing activity from optic, olfactory, gustatory, auditory and somatosensory channels are displayed on nerve cell bodies on the outermost millimeter or so of the surface of their respective cortical areas. These are the raw, minimally processed representations of perception flashing on the surface of the brain like an organic billboard. These dynamic 'pictures' on the brain are transformed, edited, and bound together with other incoming pictures.

Simultaneously, neural representations of the guitar chords from Kingdom Come, the heat on my skin, the sweat on my forehead, and the view outside my window are created while I am sitting listening to the music. They are blended together to create a multimodal picture in the higher-order association cortices. There are many such association areas, corresponding to different sensory modalities. The higher visual areas take up much more space than the primary visual cortex. In monkeys for example, more than half of the entire cerebral cortex is devoted to vision.

We can use the analogy of consciousness as something like a movie, continuously projecting ever-changing pictures as part of a coherent story. Most neuroscientists and cognitive psychologists are adamant that there is no internal 'viewer' actually sitting somewhere in the brain and watching a movie. Of course, they are right, at least in the conventional sense. I will return to the concept of the *homunculus*, or ghost in the machine later. But for now, let's continue with this useful analogy.

Reciprocating activity in the cortex and the thalamus allows cortical patterns representing things out there (sights, sounds, smells, feelings, thoughts) to reverberate temporally, and connect with similarly reverberating representations of other things out there. The thalamus is the engine or motor powering a sort of never-ending movie projector whose images play on the surface of the cerebral cortex from before birth to the moment of death. Each time a cortical pattern cycles through the thalamus over the period of several tens of milliseconds, it is subtly transformed. The integration of thousands of these transformations in time produces the illusion of motion. It is similar to the illusion created by the rapid serial succession of static images in a motion picture reel, each frame slightly different from the last.

If the thalamus is the motor of this motion picture, the higher order association cortices are the screens upon which this movie is projected. 'Looping' activity in the thalamus and cortex blends the input from various sensory modalities, but not in any haphazard way. Just as you would expect any good movie theater to project pictures that are clear and sharply focused with sound tracks that match in synch, so it is with the cinema of the mind. I hear guitar chords, feel prickly heat, and see the ripples of water in the Charles

River all at once, but I certainly don't 'hear' the heat, 'see' the chords, and 'feel' the river. There is integration with differentiation. The input is blended but not smeared.

Some people are afflicted with a curious neurological disorder called *synesthesia*. They actually (not just metaphorically) experience one sensory modality for another. Some of them become musicians who have the gift of being able to 'see the colors' of music. Others are artists who can 'hear the sounds' of a perfume or a landscape. Still others are mathematical prodigies who 'feel' numbers as we would experience emotions. Most cases of synesthesia run in families and are thus believed to be caused by genetic glitches. When geneticists pinpoint the mutations responsible for the various synesthesias, the role of these genes in the proper wiring of the brain will be better understood. Other cases may result from traumatic insults to parts of the association cortex or their connections that are important in the proper segregation of different perceptual channels.

Consciousness is not an all or nothing proposition. It is less like a binary switch than like a sunrise, slowly dawning over a landscape of oblivion. There are grades and shades of awareness and self-awareness. The lowest levels are supported by fiber tracts originating from neurons deep in the brainstem. These ascending fibers form extensive synapses with the cortex, the thalamus, and subcortical areas such as the amygdala, the hippocampus, and the basal ganglia. Together, they form the *reticular activating system* (RAS). The RAS modulates the activity of the thalamus and its circuits with the cortex. Damage to the brainstem regions housing the RAS, either deliberately inflicted on laboratory animals or resulting from strokes or motorcycle accidents in humans, causes complete loss of consciousness and coma. The modulation of cortico-thalamic activity by the RAS is necessary for awareness, but by itself it is insufficient to produce consciousness. Without reticular activation itself, an individual would be *brain-dead*, but without the rest of the brain to activate, she would be in a *persistent vegetative state*. Neither is conscious, but there is a difference. Recent advances in neuroimaging are beginning to address the ethical implications of removing such people from life support.

All this is preliminary. Recall that in my Kingdom Come reverie, I imagined that I was walking along a beach in Southern California on a hot, hazy morning. How does a real time awareness of tone sequences, prickly heat on my skin, and a view outside my window cause me to imagine something so utterly different in nature? The answer is that the visual, auditory, and somatosensory association areas, which are located primarily on the posterior parts of the brain are also wired up to four quite different systems: the motor system, the limbic system, the memory systems, and the prefrontal cortex. Each is a largely self-contained module (with submodules and sub-submodules) but they are nonetheless heavily connected with one another and with the thalamus and the RAS in both input and output directions. Perhaps the sensory input I received evoked a memory or an emotional state that in turn was associated with Southern California on a different occasion.

Motion

Motor control is organized in a top-down fashion (the reverse of sensory pathways). Here, top-down means that a pattern of neural organization is driven by a more abstract level of representation. Bottom-up means that more basic elements come together to create a higher level of representation. Just as perception flows from the bottom up, for example, in terms of vision: light>>>retina>>>optic nerve>>>lateral geniculate nucleus of the thalamus>>>primary visual cortex>>>dorsal and ventral streams, motion flows from the top down: supplementary and association motor cortex>>>basal ganglia and cerebellum>>>primary motor cortex>>>spinal cord>>>peripheral motor nerves>>>muscles>>>movement (Figure 2).

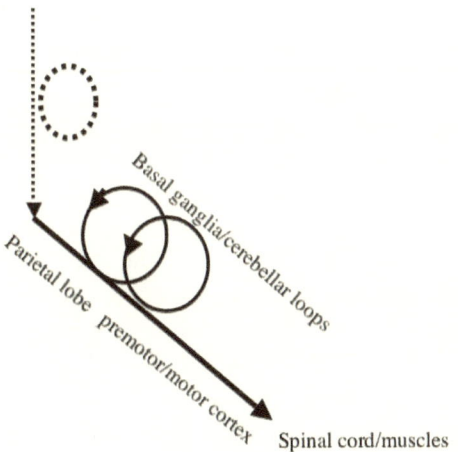

Figure 2: Motion

There is a point on this grossly simplified schematic where the highest, most abstract representations of perception are translated into the highest, most abstract representations of movement. This occurs in the frontal and parietal cortices. These regions represent information beyond simple modalities like motion, color, pain, temperature, and the coding of individual muscle movements. Rather, neurons here code for complex conjunctions of properties integrated across all the senses. The separate perceptions of sound and heat and vision are bound together into the perception of a noisy, stuffy dorm room overlooking the Charles River. They also code for the position of the perceiver's body as the reference point for these perceptions.

This last point is very important. I am using the concept of *reference frames* in terms of perception and action. Imagine playing a competitive game of tennis. You find yourself lunging forward to hit a forehand volley. There are several things going on here, each of which your brain must track simultaneously from different frames of reference. First, your legs are moving relative to the court. Second, your arm is moving relative to your body and also to the ball, which, in turn, is moving relative to the court. Third, your eyes are tracking the ball relative to the three dimensional space of the court, the motion of your head, and the motion of your body, all of which are moving relative to one another. How can you keep track of all these calculations in real time well enough to return the ball while simultaneously handling all those housekeeping activities like respiration and heartbeat? It's amazing that we can play sports at all.

It turns out that just as there are somatotopic maps of one's body image in the sensory and motor cortices, there are also body maps in the parietal cortex. These maps represent not sensations or movements of the body, but rather the 'knowledge' of one's body as the effector of action. When you decide to move your left foot, for instance, the neural command signal is given not only to the motor system, but also to the motor knowledge center in the right parietal lobe. Additionally, once you move that foot, there is a feedback signal from the muscle fibers all the way back up to this area.

The body representation maps in the parietal lobe act as thermostats tracking our intentions. Without them, we would all be bumbling klutzes. There are still other maps involved in motor control and coordination, notably in the cerebellum and the basal ganglia. These subcortical organs are responsible for automating repetitive or overlearned actions such as walking or riding a bicycle, thus freeing the cerebral cortex to attend to more demanding tasks. Damage to these subcortical regions from chronic alcoholism or Parkinson's disease causes the loss of this subconscious ability. Such patients must then *consciously* control all their motor behavior, resulting in slow, clumsy movement. On the other hand, the cortex usually exerts an inhibitory effect on subcortical automaticity centers. If subcortical motor regions are hyperactive or no longer inhibited by the cortex, as in obsessive compulsive disorder or Tourette's syndrome, motor and cognitive automaticity become uncontrollable. More on this in the next chapter.

It is in the parietal lobes that intentions are translated into action plans. Damage to the parietal lobe (usually on the left side) from a stroke or tumor leads to paralysis of the opposite side of the body, and is sometimes associated with a condition known as *anosognosia*, in which the patient denies that she even has a physical deficit. It is not that these people are so depressed or stunned by their disability that they are in denial, but rather, anosognosics actually have no idea that there is something physically wrong with their bodies! People with anosognosia can be otherwise intelligent and articulate. They understand what it means for others to be paralyzed as a result of brain damage. But they simply cannot grasp the fact that they are now unable to move one side of their own bodies. It is as if they are neglecting half of themselves. Damage to the right parietal lobe, often results in a separate, but related disorder in which the left half of the visual field is ignored. These discoveries strongly suggest that the limits of consciousness are tightly constrained by the shape of one's body image. The mind and the body really are united in more ways than one, and the proverbial 'brain in a vat' could never exist.

Emotion
Awareness of our sensory perceptions, our movements, and our bodies is usually accompanied by a certain mood. What we see and do makes us feel happy or sad or fearful or tearful. Likewise, tears and fears color our perceptions and motivate our actions. Emotions are an indelible part of the conscious experience. The *limbic system*, deep within the temporal lobe, is the emotional part of the brain. It is intimately connected both with perceptual input in the posterior cortex, and with the endocrine and the autonomic nervous systems, through the hypothalamus and the pituitary gland (Figure 3). The hypothalamus and pituitary gland control many of our bodies' homeostatic processes such as temperature regulation, sleep patterns, and general metabolic activity. We are not directly conscious or in control of these processes. But the hypothalamus also oversees our appetites for three things of which we are very conscious: food, drink, and sex.

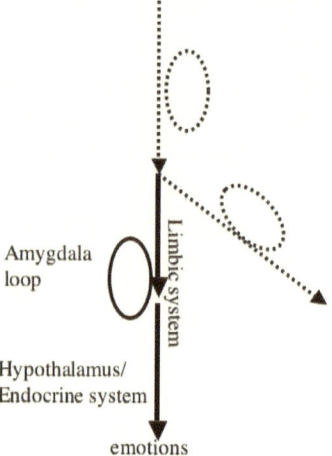

Amygdala
loop

Limbic system

Hypothalamus/
Endocrine system

emotions

Figure 3: Emotion

The heart of the limbic system is the *amygdala*. This organ has extensive connections with the hypothalamus, all the higher order sensory areas of the cerebral cortex, especially the olfactory region, the thalamus, and the parts of the temporal lobe important for long-term memory storage. The amygdala is where thoughts and perceptions acquire their *emotional valence*, which in turn helps us make better decisions. The emotional valence is kept in check by inhibitory modulation from the *prefrontal cortex* or *PFC*. An overactive amygdala (or underactive PFC) caused by temporal lobe epilepsy or massive trauma to the frontal lobe often results in impulsive, emotionally labile personality. In addition, some of these people attach great emotional significance to the mundane. Superstition, delusions of grandeur, and religious ecstasy are, as we shall see in chapter three, some of the symptoms associated with seizures in and around the amygdala.

On the other hand, an underactive amygdala (or overactive PFC) tends to dampen emotional valence. There is a rare and bizarre disorder called the *Capgras delusion* (usually caused by a blow to the head) whose sufferers come to believe that the people and places once familiar to them are not real. Capgras patients are convinced that their spouses, relatives, pets, or furniture are not who or what they seem to be, but were somehow inexplicably replaced by perfect duplicates. These people are not suffering from perceptual, memory, or cognitive impairment. They simply don't feel as if the people and things around them, especially those with emotional significance, are what they should be. It is believed that Capgras syndrome and other related depersonalization disorders are caused by disconnections in the fibers connecting the amygdala with various parts of the sensory cortex.

Memory

The feelings and emotions I got by listening to the song reminded me of a beach in Southern California. I had not been to any such beach, but I could certainly imagine it based upon my memories of other beaches and on my knowledge of the geography and climate of Southern California. Emotions are inexorably linked to memories and imagination. Experiences are converted into memory through the gateway of the *hippocampus*. This structure stores the memory trace for a period of time before it is transferred to the cortex via the thalamus, where it becomes long-term memory.

Bilateral damage to the hippocampi causes partial *retrograde amnesia* (the inability to recall information experienced or learned shortly before the injury) and *anterograde amnesia* (the inability to lay down any subsequent memories). Patients with this dreadful problem retain their personality and intelligence, but are forever trapped in their here and now. This is probably the normal state of affairs for most non-human creatures. They are fully conscious of their core selves, and of their immediate world, but in a very nearsighted way. So much of who we are as individuals depends upon a feeling of a permanent self – it requires autobiographical knowledge. This is impossible without a healthy hippocampus (Figure 4).

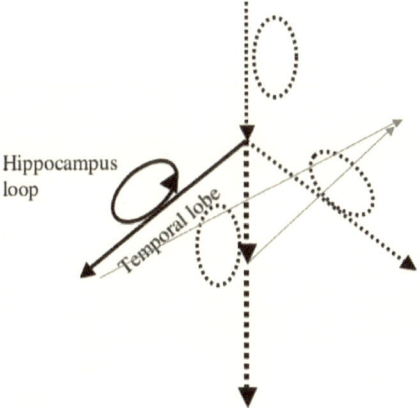

Figure 4: Memory

The emotional and memory centers of the brain (the amygdala and hippocampus) are intimately connected. Furthermore, both centers receive sensory input, especially from the olfactory system and the ventral visual stream. This is why memories so often evoke strong emotions and emotions evoke poignant memories. It is also why odors, both fragrant and obnoxious, often provoke visceral memories.

Executive Control

I have now almost completed the construction of the model mind. What remains is the integration of the sensory, motor, limbic, and memory modules through time. Although the philosopher Dan Dennett is adamant that there is no commanding homunculus that puts all these disparate activities together in some central 'Cartesian theater', I believe that a spatial-temporal integration of sorts does occur. The key players are the thalamus, the PFC, and *the anterior cingulate cortex (AC)*. The PFC, which has evolved to massive proportions in the human species, contains neural ensembles that code for goal-directed associations of sensory, motor, limbic, and mnemonic information via the neurotransmitter, *dopamine*. This is where goals are set, complex action sequences are planned, and decisions are made. Psychologists call these functions 'working memory' and 'executive control'. Damage to the PFC causes defects in working memory and executive control, as well as personality problems such as impulsiveness or indecisiveness (*Figure 5*).

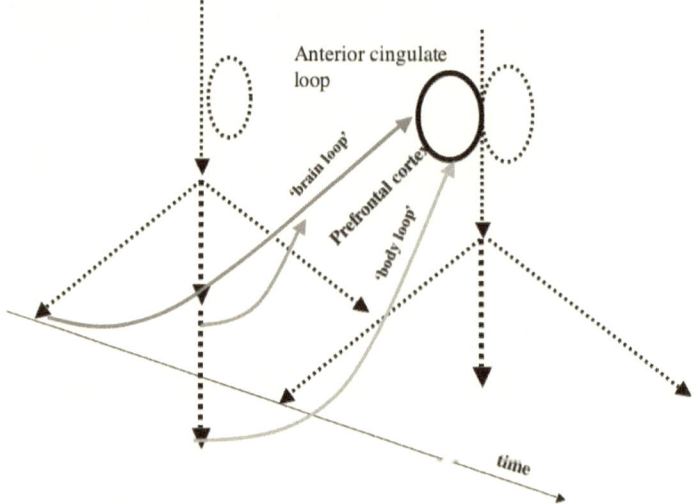

Figure 5: Executive control

Information from the PFC is fed into the AC and the thalamus. The thalamus links the goals with incoming sensory information and outgoing motor commands in a looping triangular circuit. The AC is a kind of coincidence detector that is activated by novel or conflicting input. When aroused, it sends signals into the limbic system, which in turn activates the sympathetic nervous system, heightening our sense of awareness, producing the feeling of 'SURPRISE!', and motivating further action. I believe this is where we get the sensation of 'free will'. Damage to the AC can lead to *akinetic mutism*. People with this odd disorder are neither unconscious nor comatose, but seem to lack all motivation or desire. They will sit around all day in constant ennui, gazing off into oblivion, saying nothing at all. In short, they have lost their free will.

A Model Mind

Step back and take a look at the model mind (*Figure 6*). I believe that this model, metaphorical though it is, captures something of the essence of the mind – both its modularity and its dynamic interconnections. But where exactly is consciousness, or more specifically, the P, S, and A varieties thereof, within this model?

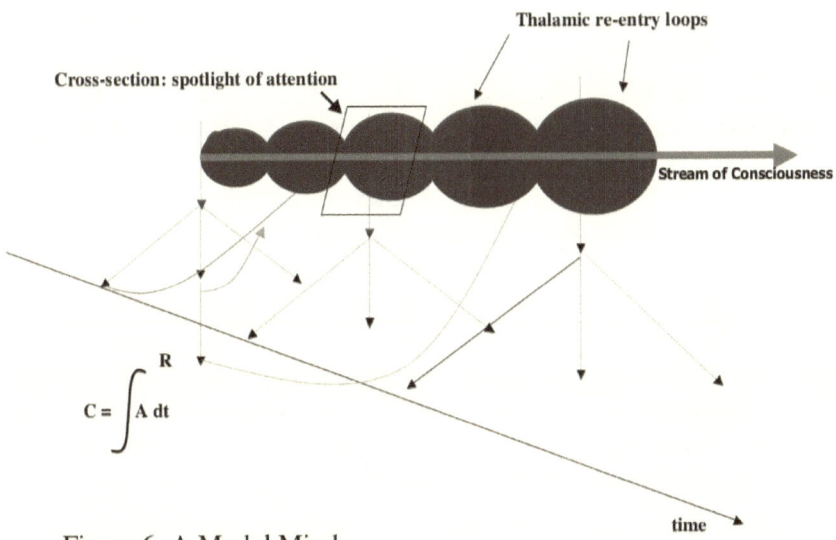

Figure 6: A Model Mind

I believe that consciousness is a continuous stream that links each of these clumsy stick figures of the mind together. Note that my mind figures have three major levels from top to bottom: 1) sensory/perceptual input, 2) cortico-thalamic reentry loops, and 3) motion/emotion/memory systems. The metaphorical stream of consciousness traverses not all three, but just the second (intermediate) level.

Before his untimely death from leukemia at age 35, the English computational neuroscientist David Marr speculated (correctly) that we are aware only of certain levels of visual processing. It is quite obvious that the lower levels, such as the shadows cast by objects reflected on the curved surface of the retina, are not reported directly to consciousness. Likewise, the high level calculations that produce the illusion of three-dimensionality are also not readily available to consciousness. Rather, it is the middle level of neurocomputation of which we are aware.

The Binding Problems Solved

My model mind makes for a nice story, but does it really explain how everything comes together? Perceptions, emotions, body images, and memories are somehow integrated into what feels like a coherent, unified self that makes decisions and strives towards goals.

The binding together of perception, motion, emotion, and memories into a continuously experienced and coherent awareness is the Holy Grail for cognitive neuroscientists. There are three separate binding problems which need to be solved separately. The first concerns the subconscious integration of various different aspects of a perceived object or event. I will call this 'perceptual binding'. The second involves the focusing of attention on a single particular integrated object or event within a field of space and time. I will call this 'attentional binding'. Finally, there is the issue of how a moving spotlight of attention is interpreted in terms of a coherent self who is able to talk about it. Let's call this 'executive binding'. I believe that solving each of the three binding problems will also give us the answer to the three most important questions in modern neuroscience: how the brain codes information (the coding problem), the neural basis for qualia (P consciousness), and the architecture of extended consciousness (S consciousness and A consciousness). Some philosophers of the mind such as Ned Block and David Chalmers argue that the first question is 'easy' while the other two questions are 'hard'. I think they have it the wrong way around. At any rate, I believe that coding problem needs to be solved rather comprehensively before we can put the others to rest. So let's get cracking!

Perceptual Binding and the Neural Code

One way of accounting for how our brains handle information would be to imagine that each and every quantum of memory, knowledge, and perception that one could conceivably experience corresponds to a specific neuron. This has been called the 'grandmother cell theory' – referring to the existence of a hypothetical neuron whose sole job it is to represent your grandmother. But a single neuron is just a stupid on-off switch; it carries only one bit of information. Therefore, you would need neurons to represent all the different perceivable aspects of your grandmother. There would be a neuron for 'a happy grandmother' or 'a sad grandmother' or 'a sad grandmother in a red polka dot dress looking forlornly out of the window of an otherwise desolate bus depot as the Milwaukee intercity pulls out into the prairies on a late sunny afternoon' (and a neuron for each and every one of those polka dots) and so on. Even given the 100 billion or so neurons and their 100 trillion synapses in a typical brain, the grandmother cell theory is quite absurd. There are simply not enough neurons or synapses in a single brain (or in all the brains in the universe!) to represent the totality of possible contingencies. The possibilities are infinite.

Rather, the brain represents objects, events, thoughts, and memories using a combinatorial system. Combinations of synapses, offering an infinite number of patterns, dynamically turning on and off throughout the brain encode all the information in our heads, both conscious and unconscious. It is not yet clear how these combinations are programmed. One idea, proposed by neuroscientist Eric Kandel of Columbia University, is that those special ascending neurons in the brainstem RAS form intimate synaptic connections with networks of cortical neurons in areas of the brain which process perceptual input. When something salient or noteworthy captures our attention, these modulatory cells fire. These connections bind together all the cortical activity that was occurring at the same time so that it is coded 'as if' it were a single discrete object or event, which is usually the case. This coincidence detector is mediated by special receptors on the neuron's synaptic membrane, called NMDA receptors, and by modulatory neurotransmitters such as serotonin and dopamine that are released by the synapses of the modulating RAS neurons. This biochemical process, which neuroscientists call *synaptic plasticity*, allows specific neurons, each corresponding to a different aspect of an object, such as its color or sound or texture or smell, to be connected within a moment of time.

There is growing evidence from several different areas of neuroscience that synaptic plasticity is the mechanism that binds subconscious contents of perception, memory, and imagination together, elevating those things above a critical threshold for subsequent conscious processing. Synaptic plasticity at the RAS/cortex interface may be necessary for this to occur, but I don't think it is sufficient by itself.

Perceptual binding involves the simultaneous activation of neuronal ensembles and their connections within the confines of the cerebral cortex. The particular unfurling geometric pattern of the ensemble network is the neural code that represents mental information. One can make a rough analogy between neural code and genetic code. Just as the secret of life is contained in the sequence of nucleotides along the one-dimensional DNA strand, the secret of the mind is contained in the activation pattern of neural connections in the three-dimensional space along the outer two millimeters of the brain surface.

We can take this analogy even further. Historically, the language of the genes was deciphered in three stages. The first happened in the late 1960's when the legendary pioneers of molecular biology like Francis Crick, Sidney Brenner, Har Gobind Korhana, and Marshall Nirenberg cracked the genetic code by determining which DNA triplet corresponded to each of the twenty physiological amino acids. The second stage was achieved a decade later, when Fred Sanger and Walter Gilbert invented a way to sequence the order of nucleotides on the DNA strand. The final triumph came in 2000 with Craig Venter and the International Consortium's announcement of the first draft of the entire human genome. With these three tremendous breakthroughs, our current understanding of the molecular basis of life is complete enough to enable us, at least in principle, to clone another human being.

We will need to do something as revolutionary for the language of the mind. There, as it was for the genetic code, three hurdles stand in our way. First, neuroscientists need to determine which neural/synaptic pattern corresponds to a particular psychological state. Second, they need to invent a way to 'image' and replicate such a three-dimensional neural ensemble. Finally, this technology needs to be improved to the point that one can 'sequence' the moving patterns of thought in real time. At that stage, our understanding of the neurological basis of psychology would be complete enough, at least in principle, to read another person's mind. While this sounds like science fiction now, so did the concept of cloning a half century ago. The technical barriers are certainly formidable, but not impossible to overcome, given the current acceleration in microprocessor speed.

Attentional Binding and the Spotlight of Attention

Cortical ensembles are the contents of thought, the stuff of consciousness. This level of integration produces moving pictures sort of like little *You Tube* videos: for example, the actress Jennifer Aniston with a line from her latest movie or a riff from Kingdom Come. There are thousands upon thousands of videos in your head, some hardly distinguishable from the next. A handful of them are full-bodied and robust, complete with surround-sound and high definition color, while others are small and grainy, and still others are just rudimentary still pictures, barely discernable to the mind's eye. Bound as they may be, one cannot be conscious of them all at once. The pictures run concurrently on parallel tracks, only one of which can enter awareness at a time. Most bound ensembles are pre-attentive and subconscious.

Attention refers to the process by which one object or event is *selected for* conscious awareness. Decades of research on attention using animals, brain damaged patients, and neuroimaging have consistently implicated one region of the brain, the *thalamus*. This paired walnut-sized subcortical organ is evolutionarily ancient, predating the surrounding cerebral cortex by several hundred million years. In all that time, it has gotten to know everybody. The thalamus is the gateway for all the senses except smell, and receives massive axonal projections from the ascending spinal cord as well as from the eyes and ears on their way up to their respective cortical areas. There are over thirty distinct thalamic nuclei (neuron clusters), each of which is intimately connected to a particular region of the cortex. Perhaps even more importantly, the thalamus receives back-projections from those very same parts of the cortex. These back and forth loops are responsible for top-down filtering or 'gating' of new information before arriving at the cortex. Neuronal loops are found throughout the brain, both within the cortex and within other subcortical organs such as the amygdala. But the cortico-thalamic loop architecture appears to be the one correlated with attention.

What exactly happens at the cortico-thalamic interface? Millions of neurons on the surface of the cerebral cortex (the gray matter) send their axons deep into the brain (the white matter) to make trillions of synapses with neurons in the thalamus. Most of these axons come from large cells called *pyramidal neurons* that are arranged in discrete *cortical columns* about two millimeters square. Each column contains several thousand neurons and over a million connections. Like nephrons in the kidney and alveoli in the lung, cortical columns are the basic functional units of the cerebral cortex.

The primary visual cortex, for example, is organized into a series of adjoining columns, each of which codes visual stimuli with a particular spatial orientation. These orientation columns are then further segregated into ocular dominance columns, which depict input from opposite eyes, and into 'hyper-columns', which process color input. Many other areas of the cortex beyond the visual areas also have well defined spatial organizations that map to some logical pattern in the outside world, such as the surface of the body. Axons from these cells all synapse on the thalamus, which, in turn, has its own corresponding maps of various different sensory, motor, or conceptual domains. The computational neuroscientist Christof Koch maintains that the matching maps on the thalamus and cortex are important in binding the representations of 'things' in the cortex with attention mediated by the thalamus, elevating these representations into conscious awareness. Sensory input from the area being attended to arrives at the thalamus and is transmitted to the corresponding region of the cortex. After processing this signal, the cortex then replies to the thalamus, via back projections, linking this sensory picture with the next one coming in.

Synchronicity

It is amazing that the billions of synapses it presumably takes to build up the representation of a concept keep their integrity through repeated trips from the cortex to thalamus and back, all while a blizzard of new information and random noise constantly reset the cortical attractors. It is as if we took a completed jigsaw puzzle, threw it off the Grand Canyon, and it landed in the Colorado River below pretty much intact. Somehow order is maintained amidst the chaos. The key lies in neural synchronicity.

Activated pyramidal neurons create a field of excitation around them, lowering the threshold at which their neighbors will fire. This facilitates synchronized firing of neighboring neurons. Because these neurons often synapse with cells many millimeters away, large zones of activity can arise. Within these zones, neural activity oscillates at different frequencies depending on what the individual is experiencing or attending to. Sleep is associated with a neural firing frequency of 12-25 cycles per second. This is known as the *beta rhythm*. Wakefulness, on the other hand, is associated with the *gamma rhythm* (25-70 cycles per second). Some neuroscientists have speculated that the gamma rhythm might be the neural correlate of conscious experience. This is supported by the fact that unconscious states such as epilepsy and deep sleep involve a slower hypersynchronization of neural activity. Additionally, altered states of consciousness, such as schizophrenic hallucinations, also seem to be associated with a loss of the gamma oscillation.

It is tempting to think of synchronized firing of large ensembles of neurons in the cortex and their counterparts in the thalamus at a certain frequency as a 'pacemaker' that drives attention and binds the components of the conscious experience against the natural tendency for disorder. The idea of oscillations acting as a kind of neural correlate of consciousness is appealing at an intuitive level, but we are still awaiting more direct evidence to support this.

Attention's Spotlight

There may not be a central focus in the brain where everything comes together in what the philosopher Dan Dennett disparagingly calls a 'Cartesian Theater'. But the way in which the parallel streams of moving mental pictures shuttle through the thalamus does create a sort of central computational bottleneck. One can make an analogy between attaining consciousness and driving your car on a multilane freeway that converges towards a single lane tunnel. As we move in towards the thalamus, those lanes progressively merge until there is a stretch through which all traffic must slow down and pass through single-file. This creates the illusion of a unitary focus of attention. It is through this focus, this 'spotlight of attention' if you will, that a coherent stream of consciousness flows. I propose that a serial stream of neural flow arising out of a massively parallel architecture will necessarily give rise to a compelling feeling of salience and subjectivity: the essence of P consciousness. Francis Crick has written about this in terms of visual attention:

'A common metaphor is that there is a 'spotlight' of visual attention. Inside the spotlight the information is processed in some special way. This makes us see the attended object or event more accurately and more quickly and also makes it easier to remember. Outside the 'spotlight' the visual information is processed less, or differently, or not at all. The attentional system of the brain moves this hypothetical spotlight rapidly from one place in the visual field to another, just as, on a slower time scale, you move your eyes.

The spotlight metaphor in its simplest form rather implies that the visual system pays attention to one *place* in the visual field. There is much indirect evidence that it does this. An alternative is that attention is paid, not to a particular place, but to a particular object. If the object moves (the eyes being kept still) then in some cases attention can be shown to be attached to the object rather than staying in one place. At the moment it seems likely that both forms of attention- to a visual object or to a visual place- can occur to some extent.'
[F. Crick, The Astonishing Hypothesis, pg. 62]

Visual awareness seems to arise from selective attention to the visual field. Without attention, visual processing still occurs through the early parts of the visual pathway from the retina through the LGN (lateral geniculate nucleus) of the thalamus, to V1, V2, and beyond. Along the way, there are modules that detect various individual features such as motion, edge orientation, brightness, color, shape from shading, even faces. But all of this parallel processing is subconscious because there is no spotlight of attention to tell 'us' what is salient. Saliency usually, though not always, involves conjunction of features. Examples include a round ball that has a certain color, shape, and motion, or a particular face that expresses a certain emotion and evokes specific memories. Parallel processors may be good at detecting individual features, but are not particularly good at calculating conjunctions. A serial search is a better strategy for that.

The contents of conscious experience, which are usually conjunctional, must first pass through a serial processor that focuses attention on specific combinations of features. This is where those cortico-thalamic loops come in. Parallel processors outside these loops perform pre-attentive, subconscious computations, but serial processors embodied by the loops perform attentive, conscious ones.

*****

There is a distinction between the *process* of attentional binding and the *contents* of phenomenal consciousness. Thalamic neurons and their cortical counterparts are largely hardwired at birth. Developmental geneticist Carla Shatz has found that retinal neurons in embryonic mice send their fibers to their proper targets in the cortex even in the absence of light. The extent of experience-driven plasticity, while remarkable, has its limits. Mirganka Sur's now classic experiments in re-wiring the optical and auditory pathways in fetal ferret cortex probably produced more brain damage than true synesthesia. Thanks to the very nature of their connections, the cortico-thalamic loops inside every infant's brain are pre-programmed for attention long before they attend to anything at all.

On the other hand, the process by which cortical ensembles are selected for attention is Darwinian. A Darwinian process simply involves the replication of patterns with slight variation and the competition of these patterns for selection to the next round. It is not limited to sexually mature creatures or to molecules of DNA. The selection of antibodies in the immune system is another example. If we ever succeed in producing artificial intelligence or discover extraterrestrial intelligence, its evolution too will likely be governed by Darwinian processes that have nothing to do with genes or immunoglobulins or DNA. As we shall see later, neuroscientists have come up with models of consciousness by applying the robust principles of Darwinian selection to the patterns of neural activity within those integrated cortical loops.

At the cellular level, the competition for entry into the charmed circle of attention is fierce. Coalitions of neurons and their associated three-dimensional fiber patterns constantly jostle with one another for access to the proper thalamic oscillation frequency. To become successful, a winning coalition must 'take over' more thalamic connections (perhaps by reaching a certain net electrochemical threshold?) than any of the thousands of other ensembles currently up for consideration back in the cortex. Once a coalition is in power, there may be some mechanisms such as positive feedback loops that allow it to stay within the spotlight. But the competition never lets up and rival ensembles are always lurking in the shadows.

I propose a plausible neuronal mechanism for the selection of a cortical pattern for entry into the spotlight of attention. Imagine three cortical ensembles **A**, **B**, and **C** representing three discrete objects or events, for example the actress *Jennifer Aniston*, the *Taj Mahal*, and an *itch on your nose*, respectively (**Figure 7**). Each ensemble is physically unique, although they may share some common nodes. Imagine another set of three ensembles **a**, **b**, and **c** representing neuron groups in the thalamus, each of which has dedicated reciprocal connections with the corresponding cortical neuron groups **A**, **B**, and **C**. At times when one is not thinking of Jennifer Aniston, the Taj Mahal, or one's itchy nose, none of the cortical ensembles are activated, and therefore no cortico-thalamic loops are occupied. In situations where cortical pattern **A** is activated, the corresponding thalamic pattern **a** will necessarily fire. This initiates cortico-thalamic oscillations **A/a** within the circle of attention that lead to an awareness of Jennifer Aniston. In addition, the activation of the **A/a** loop may simultaneously inhibit the potential of other loops within a certain time frame. Finally, let's take a case where **A**, **B**, and **C** are all activated at the same time, but **C** happens to be the most salient. Perhaps you're talking to your roommate about how fabulous a trip to India would be while watching an episode of 'Friends', when you suddenly experience an intense itch on your nose. Here, three separate loops **A/a**, **B/b**, and **C/c** may be engaged all at once. But in this case **C** is the ensemble with the largest 'penumbra' (the set of cortical neurons with access to **C**, but not to **A** or **B**). So **C** tends to be more depolarized than **A** or **B**. As a result, the contents of the **C/c** loop is currently displayed in consciousness, while the other two loops keep spinning around in the subconscious, waiting to be drawn in. In this case, we are talking about the neural correlate of an itchy nose.

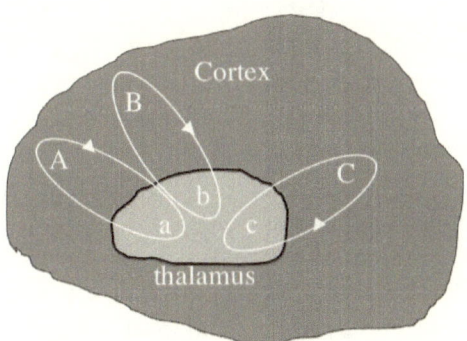

Figure 7: cortico-thalamic loops

Dan Dennett believes that the myriad contents of our conscious lives simply seem to form a continuous thread because those neural patterns representing objects or events that are most similar or complementary to other things already in mind are biased and recruited into the spotlight of attention where they can spawn more such patterns. On the other hand, patterns that represent random unrelated things become extinct. Chosen patterns tend to stabilize and stay in the spotlight because they attract like-minded patterns. Examples include 'light and warmth', 'macaroni and cheese', 'fishnets and garter belts', or 'crime and punishment'. The strength of these relationships is determined by the usefulness of the association for the survival and reproductive success of the individual hosting these neural patterns. Once a successful consortium of associated neural patterns representing a useful behavior or thought emerges, it tends to survive and stay on in the mind as a stable cluster.

But what happens *outside* the spotlight of attention? Parallel processing of sensory, emotional, mnemonic, imaginary, and other mental information undoubtedly occurs, but the results usually remain hidden from conscious access. Sometimes, however, these subconscious processes bubble up to the surface. The phenomenon of *blindsight*, discovered by the English psychologist Lawrence Weiskrantz, is one example. People who have suffered strokes to the primary visual cortex are effectively blind over the corresponding field of vision. When shown a stimulus within their *scotoma* (blind spot), they report seeing nothing. Yet when experimenters persistently prompt them to guess where this invisible object is, they often 'guess' correctly more often than chance should allow! It turns out that there are visual pathways from the retina to the *superior colliculus*, a subcortical brain structure used to orient eye movements. These subcortical pathways bypass the thalamus and are therefore not part of conscious awareness; yet they can play a small role in guiding our behavior. Incidentally, in some lower animals such as frogs, the collicular visual pathway is the major route from eye to brain. Collicular neurons are sensitive to movements only. This is why frogs are so good at catching flies in midair, but would starve to death if put in a tank with dead flies. In such creatures, all sight is 'blindsight'.

Alternatively, things that should normally stay safely inside the charmed circle of attention sometimes fall out. This occurs in *hemispatial neglect* (usually caused by a stroke in the right parietal lobe) where the left half of the visual field, or sometimes even the left half of objects in either field are lost from conscious awareness. The right parietal lobe orients attention to a particular frame of reference. Damage here prevents the spotlight from shining on the left visual field.

Balint's syndrome, caused by bilateral damage to the occipital/parietal regions, interferes with the ability to focus attention on more than one object at a time. When such patients are shown an array of red and green circles and asked to name the color, they pick the color of the object upon which they happen to focus attention. The other objects are neglected because the dorsal stream, which locates objects in space, is knocked out.

Even in 'normal' people, most of what we see cannot be inside the spotlight all at once. Attention works serially. We can experience and describe whatever is within the spotlight, but have a very foggy idea about what is not. This explains why the perceptual features of unattended objects, for example, things seen out of the corner of the eye or our recollection of the colors of people's clothing after a cursory glance, often smear into vagueness.

In summary, attention and consciousness require some but not all cortical regions. These include the various parts of the primary and higher-order sensory cortex where the contents of consciousness reside, and the parietal lobe, which orients attention to them. While potentially conscious neural ensembles can be found almost anywhere in the cortex at any given time, only a small region of the cortex will actually achieve consciousness. Attention does requires the thalamus, which generates the spotlight of attention. However, none of the other important subcortical structures, such as the amygdala, hippocampus, and basal ganglia, are absolutely necessary for consciousness.

As I explained earlier, attention refers to the process by which a series of cortical ensembles representing an object, event, body state, feeling, image, or memory is selected by and shunted back and forth through the thalamus, acquiring a richness of texture and depth of character lacking in cortical ensembles that are not so chosen. While attention is necessary and sufficient for phenomenal/core consciousness, it is insufficient for extended/verbal access and self-consciousness.

The neural architecture of the cortico-thalamic loop constrains attention and consciousness to a single channel. In principle, the content of each functioning loop is conscious. The fact that most of us are usually aware of a single stream of thought at a time indicates that only one loop can be selected at once. An unusual exception may be the case of *split-brain patients*; more on that later. The process of attention shines a roving spotlight on a single conscious stream as it flows amidst many unattended subconscious channels.

Recent studies have shown that the process of awareness occurs serially on top of distributed parallel circuits, which would explain the temporal and spatial resource limitations of attentive search tasks. The psychologist Anne Treisman has done some seminal research on this:

> 'Some features of surfaces and depth can be detected without focusing attention: thus, parallel detection is possible for properties defined by stereoscopic depth, constancy scaling

of brightness, and geometric forms seen as three-dimensional objects lit from a particular direction. These properties conjoin many simple retinal cues, in apparent conflict with the claim that serial attention is needed for binding. One resolution is that parallel search reflects not pre-attentive processing but global attention to the scene as a whole, with no individuation of separate elements. A discrepant object is seen as a break in the global structure of the three-dimensional array. Similarly, a face can be seen as a global whole without requiring serial processing of each feature in turn...Conjunctions of parts may create emergent features, such as closure, which also allow parallel detection. Extensive practice may form new conjunction detectors that mediate efficient search, suggesting the possibility that 'grandmother cells' or local 'cell assemblies' may develop to solve the binding problem for familiar sets of items such as letters, or for useful components of more complex shapes...Recent evidence continues to support the idea that binding depends on attention unless one or other of these special conditions holds.' [Treisman, A, 1996, 'The binding problem', <u>Current Opinion in Neurobiology</u>]

The results of psychological experiments designed to erase or tease out the distinction between parallel/pre-attentive and serial/attentive processing have been somewhat contradictory. Treisman's classic studies on visual search demonstrated that picking out a unique target among a field of distracters (for instance, a red 'T' surrounded by blue 'T's and 'O's) involves a 'pop-out' or parallel search, while selecting a target hidden in a field of distracters with some features in common (a red 'T' among red 'O's and blue 'T's) requires a longer conjunction or serial search. While it seems clear that conjunction searches require conscious attentive effort, it does not follow that pop-out searches are necessarily pre-attentive and unconscious. It is quite possible that the contents of multiple parallel neural traces (the target and the distracters in the pop-out search above) can all enter the spotlight at the same time, as parts of a larger unified and coherent 'picture', so long as processing demands are not overloaded. This was the position taken by Francis Crick and Christof Koch in a paper published shortly before Crick's death at age 88:

'Several objects/events can be handled simultaneously – more than one object/event can be attended to at the same time – if there is no significant overlap in any cortical neural network.

That is, if two or more objects/events do not have any very active essential nodes in common, they can be consciously perceived. Under such conditions, several largely separate (sensory) coalitions may exist. If there is necessarily such an overlap, then (top-down) attention is needed to select one of them by biasing the competition among them.' [F. Crick & C. Koch, 2003, 'A Framework for Consciousness', <u>Nature Neuroscience</u>]

*****

The spotlight of attention is constantly moving around a 'global workspace', illuminating swaths of the subconscious landscape one stretch at a time. The contents of attention are kept in short term memory and constantly compared with refreshed versions, as the cortico-thalamic circuit traverses newly re-entering loops. Because we remember the contents of the previously attended location, the ever-fleeting spotlight's trace is experienced not as choppy snapshots, but rather as a continuous and coherent moving picture of the world. Moreover, our ambient emotions and memories color this illusory movie all the while.

The action of the loops creates a perceptual moment in our center of attention, and the movement of that center through time produces continuous experience. If the spotlight were to stop moving and fixate on only one object, perhaps as a result of damage to the thalamus or parietal lobe (those regions responsible for shifting attention from place to place), then our conscious awareness of the spotlight's contents would be lost as well.

One can make an analogy with the rapid eye movements we all make whilst awake. Our vision is concentrated on the fifteen or so degrees of space reflected on our foveae. The remainder of the world is either invisible (because our eyes don't see it) or barely visible (through peripheral vision) or subconsciously visible (through blindsight). Yet we do not experience the world as if looking through a peephole. Each waking second, our eyes make three to five involuntary movements called *saccades*. Saccades function to stimulate the retinal cells with continuous fresh visual input that provides useful updates of the outside world. Like all neurons, retinal ganglion cells are activated not by the absolute magnitude of the perceived stimulus, but rather by *relative changes* in contrast over time. If the eyes failed to saccade, there would be no change in contrast and so the picture in the mind's eye would gradually fade to black. Saccades produce the illusion of visual continuity by moving the 'ocular spotlight' around to create a seamless ribbon of visual experience. Likewise, attention shifting produces the illusion of subjective continuity by moving the 'attentional spotlight' around to create a seamless ribbon of conscious experience.

*****

I would like to close the gap between attention and consciousness. Let's quickly review what happens. First, neurons in your brainstem activating system set up synchronized gamma oscillations in your thalamus and cerebral cortex. This is what is generally referred to as being awake. Second, this synchronicity automatically attracts cortical patterns coding for an endless assortment of possible objects, events, thoughts, memories, ideas, and emotions. A particular pattern is selected for attention if it has a large enough penumbra. The pattern within this loop is now within the 'spotlight of attention.' Third, subconscious neural traces recruited into the spotlight traverse the loop several times a second, losing or gaining strength each time. Eventually, new sensations allow other coalitions of cortical patterns to take over. This is how the mind drifts when you think about something else. Attention is simply whatever pattern happens to be twirling around the loop at a given time. I should emphasize here that nothing physically moves around in a circle. Rather, I am simply using a metaphor referring to a specific pattern of electrical signals in one part of the brain causing a different pattern of electrical signals in another part of the brain.

Finally, consciousness, unlike the spotlight of attention, is not a near instantaneous snapshot, but rather an ongoing process. Despite how we may feel about it, the conscious moment does not exist at an absolute point in time; it is instead constructed from comparisons to representations stored in various parts of the brain. It involves the continuous summation of slices of attention as the spotlight moves serially from thought to thought, illuminating different people, places, events, feelings, and memories all the while. In other words, consciousness is simply the *integration* of the contents of the spotlight of attention as it traverses re-entrant cortico-thalamic loops through time. The repetitive, iterative nature of this mechanism creates the depth and thickness of our experienced reality. One is tempted to express this mathematically with a few simple equations in which **A** is attention, **E** is cortical ensemble, **R** is the area of re-entry, and **C** is consciousness:

$$\mathbf{A} = \mathbf{E} \times \mathbf{R}$$
and
$$\mathbf{C} = \sum \mathbf{A} \text{ over time}$$
or

$$C = \int A dt$$

In truth, things get messy. The definition of integration implies the averaging of constituents; if we summate and average slices of attention, we would end up with an undifferentiated smear. It is more accurate to say that there is both integration (of the attentional stream) into a coherent story, as well as a differentiation (of the various components being attended to). How can both be true? Perhaps it is too naïve to describe the phenomenology of consciousness in terms of neat mathematical equations. That approach has served physicists and chemists well, but biologists and neuroscientists have always been grounded in the muck of empiricism. However, I think my model mind and consciousness equations are good metaphors for understanding the roots of thought. Allow me to take you on a tour of my magical sculpture garden (Figure 6).

The framework of the structure sitting atop the grassy knoll represents the entire mental landscape, most of it subconscious. These include incoming sensory information converging up into the thalamus, outgoing motor patterns passing down through basal ganglia and cerebellum, the amygdala encoding emotional valance onto the hypothalamus and frontal cortex, memory traces being transferred from hippocampus to temporal lobe, and so on. Consciousness is but a small part of that edifice: the looping cylinder connecting the thalamus of the past to cortex of the present to thalamus of the future and so on and on throughout the duration of a mental lifetime. The circular area inside a slice of that cylinder – the differentiated spotlight of attention at a given perceptual instant – is the consciously-remembered present. Simply put, that is phenomenal consciousness. But the richness of human consciousness owes almost everything to the memories of a lifetime and to the expectations and dreams of imagined futures. While that richness is also embedded into the conscious moment, it is only made possible by integrating that slice of attention with other slices in the past and potential slices in the future. So consciousness is necessarily both a differentiated two-dimensional circle as well as an integrated three-dimensional cylinder depending on how one examines a model mind in terms of the fourth dimension of time.

I want to briefly mention a recent theory advanced by the French neuroscientist Stanislas Dehaene. He has done some impressive work looking for the 'neural signature' of conscious perception in terms of quantifiable differences in brain activation patterns, as measured by fMRI and magnetoencepholography. His subjects were tested while they were presented with visual stimuli that were presented too quickly for conscious registration (masked stimuli) versus those which were subjectively reported with confidence (conscious stimuli). The trick is that the masked stimuli still make it into the visual areas of the brain, even up to the higher cortex, despite the subjects' denial that they saw anything at all. Recall the case of blindsight. What he found was that while both kinds of stimuli are processed by and activate the same brain regions, such as thalamus, V1, the ventral stream, limbic system, hippocampus, and so on, the effect was transient (less than a second) with the masked stimuli. For a perception to pass the threshold of conscious access, it needs to cause a reverberation throughout many parts of the brain that can be sustained indefinitely. Dehaene believes that synchronized oscillations in the gamma frequency originating from the thalamus might be the glue that elevates subconscious patterns into a 'global neuronal workspace' that can then be accessed by remote regions of the brain.

Dehaene's theory fits in nicely with Bernard Baars's idea that attention's spotlight illuminates a *global workspace* whose contents are conscious. Both are compatible with Crick and Koch's notion that consciousness happens when a percept activates enough neurons in its penumbra to set off synchronized oscillations throughout the brain. In contrast, Ann Treisman's latest research in this area suggests that another defining feature of consciousness in addition to duration is the *reproducibility* of its neural pattern across different instances of the same percept. But this is not incompatible with the Global Neuronal Workspace model if we understand that once a stable temporal-spatial workspace is set up, then different brain regions with distinct properties can all act on the same perception in their separate ways.

Executive Binding and the Nature of the Self

What we now have is a single movie playing inside a mental multiplex. The frames of the movie are bound together by synchronized oscillations of linked neural ensembles. I believe the model is still incomplete because no matter how hard we look, all we see are scintillating patterns of neural activity. But consciousness implies a certain salience to our experiences, a coherent reference point in terms of subject and object. We are aware of ourselves as a focus, a single point of reference around which all our perceptions, motions, emotions, imaginations, and memories revolve. *But where am I in all of this?*

I AM AN ILLUSION.

At the core of the model is the loop created by the reentrant spotlight of attention. As the parallel processors in various parts of the brain do their thing, the spotlight etches out a single stream of consciousness. The focus of attention shifts constantly; the intensity and size of the spotlight itself will change depending on motivation, energy, and distractions. But this stream of consciousness is what creates the sense of self. My mind is simply all that *I* am. Douglas Hofstadter points out that self-awareness can create consciousness in a mathematical system as well as a brain:

> '...the Godelian strange loop that arises in formal systems in mathematics (i.e. collections of rules for churning out an endless series of mathematical truths solely by mechanical symbol-shunting without any regard to meanings or ideas hidden in the shapes being manipulated) is a loop that allows such a system to 'perceive itself', to talk about itself, to become 'self-aware', and in a sense it would not be going too far to say that by virtue of having such a loop a formal system *acquires a self.*
>
> 'When and only when such a loop arises in a brain or in any other substrate, is a *person* – a unique new 'I' brought into being. Moreover, the more self referentially rich such a loop is, the more conscious is the self to which it gives rise. Yes, shocking though this might sound, consciousness is not an on/off phenomenon, but admits of degrees, grades, shades. Or, to put it more bluntly, there are bigger souls and smaller souls.' [Hofstadter, Gödel, Escher, Bach: An Eternal Golden Braid]

The contents of phenomenal consciousness are whatever happens to lie within the charmed spotlight of attention. The possibilities are endless: anything that we can possibly perceive, remember, or imagine is fair game. But at the same time we feel as if our conscious experience belongs to a unitary self anchored within a physical universe: the *me* that is conscious. The coherence of the stream of consciousness is yet another illusion created by a Darwinian process.

Dan Dennett maintains that serial collections of successful neural patterns – what the evolutionary biologist Richard Dawkins dubbed 'memes'

– illuminated within the spotlight of attention comprise 'multiple drafts' of an ongoing personal narrative. This narrative slowly emerges in early childhood and continues until death (or at least late senility) with regular breaks for nonREM sleep and occasionally unexpected breaks due to seizures or bumps on the head. Here are some revealing passages from his influential work, Consciousness Explained (1991):

> 'There is no single, definitive 'stream of consciousness', because there is no central Headquarters, no Cartesian Theater where 'it all comes together' for the perusal of a Central Meaner. Instead of such a single stream (however wide), there are multiple channels in which specialist circuits try, in parallel pandemoniums, to do their various things, creating Multiple Drafts as they go. Most of these fragmentary drafts of 'narrative' play short-lived roles in the modulation of current activity but some get promoted to further functional roles, in swift succession, by the activity of a virtual machine in the brain. The seriality of this machine is not a 'hard-wired' design feature, but rather the upshot of a succession of coalitions of these specialists.' [Dennett, pg 224]

> 'According to our sketch, there is competition among many concurrent contentful events in the brain, and a select subset of such events 'win'. That is, they manage to spawn continuing effects of various sorts. Some, uniting with language-demons, contribute to subsequent sayings, both sayings-aloud to others and silent (and out-loud) sayings to oneself. Some lend their content to other forms of subsequent self-stimulation, such as diagramming-to-oneself. The rest die out almost immediately, leaving only faint traces – circumstantial evidence – that they ever occurred at all.' [Dennett pg 275]

Dennett makes two other important points. First, not just verbal access and self-awareness (A and S consciousnesses), but also the very quality of the perceptual moment – William James's 'pungency of experience' or P consciousness – is itself an emergent property, an epiphenomenon arising from the deeper structures and patterns of neural computation and molecular biology. He believes that if and when we understand all the nuances of these deeper levels, 'qualia', that raw feel of first person experiences, will simply evaporate much as the concept of a vital life force lost support after the discovery of the structure of DNA.

Secondly, Dennett emphatically maintains that there is no central brain region where the stream of consciousness comes together. He dismisses the idea of the 'Cartesian Theater' and has the audacity of accusing, of all people, Francis Crick of supporting it.

*****

Let's say you and I come across a patch of violets while taking a walk in the garden. I point out to you how lovely those violets look and you agree. Because both of us describe the flowers in the same words, and each of us believes the other has seen the same thing. But is this true? Is the violet that I see the same as the violet that you see? Words alone cannot make it so; I cannot know for sure without stepping into your mind.

We don't have to go that far. The truth is that the first person subjective experience of anything (the scent of a flower, a bar of music, the view of a sunset) is never exactly the same for another person because it is necessarily imbued with emotions and memories unique to that individual. The perceived moment is an interpretation that has already been through several layers of editing before reaching consciousness, and no two people, not even identical twins, have the same team of editors. Furthermore, it seems clear to me that even a single individual never experiences something the same way twice. My experienced qualia are influenced by extrinsic factors such as mood, motivation, and memories. But they are also determined by the genes that control the way our neurons get wired up during development. Nature and nurture conspire to make every experience feel different not just for any two people, but also for any one person on two different occasions.

I disagree with Dennett's final point. Attention is bound and consciousness expressed in several key areas of the brain. There are, in fact, many Cartesian Theaters playing nearby. In their search for the NCC, researchers have uncovered several brain areas that are likely to be very important for the binding of subjective conscious experiences. Francis Crick believes that the PFC, the thalamus, and the anterior cingulate gyrus are essential for consciousness. Vilayanur Ramachandran, on the other hand, believes that the temporal lobe is the site where awareness happens. Perhaps they are both right.

Philosophers and sages have long remarked on the compelling sense one has of oneself as a unitary entity that endures over time and circumstance. So profound is this feeling that throughout the centuries otherwise reasonable people have been compelled to believe that 'the self' can somehow survive the physical destruction of its body. Largely from this irrational belief arose all those crazy myths of reincarnation and spirituality (which we shall discuss in more detail in chapter three). But most of us are at least capable of entertaining the possibility that this might all be a big illusion. We say this all the time: 'my, you've changed,' 'Aunt Mildred hasn't been herself lately,' 'I've just lost myself,' 'I don't know you anymore,' and so on. One could argue that, at least in physical and physiological terms, one's identity changes every few seconds. The conflict between continuity and transformation lies at the core of the seemingly unbridgeable gulf between an objective scientific inquiry of consciousness and the subjective phenomenology of self. As long as this explanatory gap remains, the 'hard problem' of consciousness will continue to seem hard.

For these sorts of problems, it's always a good idea to take the evolutionary perspective. The German philosopher Thomas Metzinger has been thinking long and hard about why we have and perhaps have a need for the illusion of self:

> 'Scientific representations of the world, and of consciousness, aim at maximal objectivity, at being very parsimonious, at not introducing superfluous entities, and at making good predictions. Phenomenal representations are clever in a different way because they had a completely different purpose: they were needed to help our parents and grandparents and all our ancestors to survive and copy their genes. Their target was not to generate a faithful representation of reality or of the brain, or the way we sensorily perceive the world; they had a completely different goal, and certain illusions can be functionally adequate- as philosophers say of misrepresentations: the belief in your own existence as a distinct self or, to say something more provocative, the belief that life is actually worth living, can be very successful in copying genes.'

> 'There is an internal image of yourself that you cannot recognize as an image while it is there – and the unromantic part is in regarding this as a weapon that emerged in the cause of the cognitive arms race. There was constant competition among organisms on this planet, for millions of years, and it was merciless and cruel and the developments of things like memory, thought, better perceptions, was just as important as better legs, better livers, better hearts. I like to look at the human self-model as a neurocomputational

weapon, a certain data structure that the brain can activate from time to time, such as when you have to wake up in the morning and integrate your sensory perceptions with your motor beahviour. The ego machine just turns on its phenomenal self, and that is the moment when *you* come to.'
[T. Metzinger interview from S. Blackmore, <u>Conversations on Consciousness</u>]

Cognitive scientists have now located Metzinger's 'ego machine'. It lies in the left hemisphere. But first some basic neuroscience.

Left and Right

The vertebrate brain is divided into left and right hemispheres separated by a massive fiber tract, the corpus callosum. In humans, the two hemispheres are nearly identical anatomically, with each hemisphere largely responsible for sensory and motor function in the opposite side of the body. However, not all is symmetrical. For example, a landmark known as the sylvian fissure is generally longer and straighter on the left side. A part of the temporal lobe called the planum temporale, which is believed to be involved in language processing, tends to be larger on the left side. The left brain is specialized for language in approximately 95% of right-handers and 70% of left-handers.

The root causes of the asymmetry lie in evolutionary and developmental processes. Brain asymmetries in mammals are related to left-right axis determination in the developing embryo, which is specified by a developmental gene called nodal. The protein products of this gene are responsible for setting up the left-right polarity in the organization of internal organs such as the heart, liver, and spleen, and also exert an influence on aspects of brain development.

Michael Corballis, a psychologist from New Zealand, believes that differences in human brain polarity arose in our primate ancestors once they started to walk upright. According to this view, bipedalism freed the arms from the symmetrical locomotion of quadrupeds, an activity likely to be best controlled by symmetrically organized hemispheres. Upright stance, however, allows specialized hand activity such as making flint tools by holding a stone in one hand while striking it with the other hand. Success in this activity clearly requires the two hands to make different movements. Thus evolutionary pressure was exerted on the brain to capitalize on any possible preexisting asymmetries to provide an efficient system for specialized hand movements. The left hemisphere seems to have been slightly better equipped to handle such complex sequential actions as tool making.

Thousands of generations of natural selection may have magnified this left-right asymmetry between the time of the first tool builders, Australopithecus africanus three and a half million years ago, and the emergence of language in modern humans about 100,000 years ago. By this time, the asymmetry was more pronounced than in non-human primates that do not use tools. Possibly because the left hemisphere became more specialized for complex movements like tool making, early hominids were more likely to be right-handed. Increased right-handed use, in turn, may have selected for further left hemisphere specialization in a kind of feedback loop. Although we cannot be sure of the causal or even temporal relationship of handedness and 'brainedness', the fossil evidence does seem to support right hand dominance in most of our ancestors.

The subsequent emergence of symbolic language produced much greater selection pressure on the left hemisphere. Spoken or gestured language is in some ways quite similar to tool making. At a physical level, the production of language involves sequential movements of the small muscles of the hands, face, tongue, and larynx. Unlike tool making, however, the motor actions associated with language production are very complex and require precise coordination. The resulting selective pressure must have been simply explosive, snowballing into the type of functional and possibly anatomic hemispheric asymmetry we find in humans today.

This idea fits nicely with studies that found differing perceptual sensitivities to high and low frequency visual stimuli selectively directed to the two hemispheres. Using normal subjects, psychologist Fred Kitterle briefly flashed images of sinusoidal gratings (horizontal stripes) of differing spatial frequency to either the left or right visual field and measured reaction times for the detection and identification of stimuli [Kitterle, F., Christman, S., and Hellige, J. (1990) 'Hemispheric differences are found in identification, but not detection of low versus high spatial frequencies'. Percept. Psychophysics 48:297-306]. He found that there was a significant time difference for the identification of wide versus narrow gratings, depending on which hemisphere received the stimuli. The right hemisphere was faster for identifying low frequency stimuli (wide gratings) presented to its visual field (the left) while the left hemisphere was faster for high frequency stimuli (narrow gratings) presented to the right visual field.

In short, the right hemisphere appears to be specialized for relatively coarse, global perception, while the left hemisphere is better at fine grain, local perception. Gist comes from the right side, fine detail from the left. Remarkably, this so-called 'frequency hypothesis' of hemispherical specialization apparently exists in auditory perception as well. Neuropsychologist Diana

Deutsch has found that the left hemisphere is better at the detection of high frequency sounds, while the right hemisphere is better able to detect sounds of low frequency [Deutsch, D. (1985). 'Dichotic listening to melodic patterns and its relationship to hemispheric specialization of function'. Music Percep.3:127-154].

A possible mechanism for the different processing patterns of the two cerebral hemispheres may lie in their differing maturation rates. Studies of embryos and infants seem to suggest that the left hemisphere matures later than the right. The delay in left hemisphere development may be related to prenatal exposure to the male sex hormone, testosterone [Geschwind, N, and Galaburda, A.M. (1987) Cerebral Lateralization: Biological Mechanisms, Associations, and Pathology]. Testosterone and other androgens have a delaying effect on the growth and maturation of the left hemisphere. The higher testosterone concentration in male fetuses tends to prolong the critical growth phase of their left hemisphere, increasing both their vulnerability to developmental insults and the likelihood of becoming right brain dominant (and left-handed). If this is true, then it implies that cognitive processes centered more on the left hemisphere may also have a longer or delayed developmental period, compared to those centered on the right.

There is a hackneyed saying in neuroscience: 'neurons that fire together, wire together.' The developing nervous system allows for input-dependent wiring or plasticity during critical maturation periods. Stimulation of immature nerve cells by external or internal stimuli during development produces the sprouting of new connections. If the left hemisphere has a longer maturation period than the right from the prenatal stage through infancy and beyond, the wiring of its circuits will reflect stimuli received at a later stage. Perhaps the right brain is more sensitive to low frequency, low resolution stimuli because that is the type of environment (in utero and early infancy) in which the infant's brain matures. In contrast, the left brain, with its delayed maturation period, will tend to receive richer, more specialized visual, auditory and other input from the infant's better developed eyes and ears, and from its more complex post-natal environment. So here we see the snowball effect at work again, this time in terms of developmental biology rather than evolution. Minor differences in laterality as programmed by our genes, and reflected in differential maturation rates, form the substrate for functional specialization in areas as disparate as perceptual frequency discrimination, tool making, and language.

These left-right differences in frequency discrimination also lead to differences in the type of coherence each hemisphere brings to our perceptions. Coherence can arise at a relatively local level when the perception is biased towards higher frequency, high-resolution sensitivity. This 'local coherence' tends to occur in the left hemisphere. In contrast, coherence can arise at a more global, holistic level, if perception occurs at a lower resolution. This is 'central coherence', and it happens in the right hemisphere.

Central coherence and local coherence are contrasting styles of cognitive integration, different ways of binding percepts and concepts together. One can say these styles run along a continuum from left brain to right brain. Both hemispheres are fully capable of most tasks. Moreover, in normal people, the two sides talk to each other all the time through the long white matter tracts of the corpus callosum. However, there are differences in processing style that can be unmasked in certain very abnormal conditions.

The Interpreter

Starting in the 1940's, neurosurgeons began to practice a radical new treatment for intractable epilepsy. In an effort to isolate the foci of these patients' terrible convulsions, these medical pioneers sliced the two cerebral hemispheres apart in a procedure known as a callosectomy. These 'split-brain' operations were a great success. Not only were the patients largely cured of their seizures; they didn't seem to suffer any untoward side effects. Their perceptions, motor control, emotional responses, memory, and judgment seemed intact. Curiously, they did seem to acquire the habit of turning their heads to the left when presented with stimuli in their left periphery, while objects in their right visual field didn't usually elicit the same degree of head-turning to the right. In the 1960's, a few neuroscientists, including Roger Sperry and his graduate student Michael Gazzaniga, began to suspect something very strange was going on behind this seemingly minor finding. They were about to make one of the seminal discoveries in the history of cognitive neuroscience.

Recall that all visual input from the right visual field goes to the left hemisphere and vice versa. Only after being processed from bottom-up to higher levels in the dorsal and ventral streams of their respective hemispheres does this information become available to the other side via the intact corpus callosum. If both hemispheres of the split brain patients needed access to visual input, then one would expect an equal amount of attention (and head-turning) to both sides. So why the bias to the left? First of all, it turns out that the left brain attends only to the right visual field while the right brain attends to the entire visual field. The corollary is that the entire brain can focus attention on an object on the right side, while only the right brain can attend to an object on the left side. Normally, this doesn't matter much because of attentional crosstalk through the callosum. But in the split-brain patient, information is segregated all the way through. In this case, the left hemisphere seems to need access to its missing information (in the left visual field) more than the right hemisphere needs access to its missing information (in the right visual field). It is almost as if the right brain can't be bothered by its lack of knowledge, while the left brain actively seeks it out.

Over the next decades, Sperry and Gazzaniga proceeded to carry out a series of novel experiments on their split-brain patients. Among their bizarre findings was that the left-brain fabricates explanations for the actions of the right brain that it doesn't know about. In Gazzaniga's own words:

> 'We showed a split-brain patient two pictures: a chicken claw was shown to his right visual field, so the left hemisphere saw only that, and a snow scene was shown to the left visual field, so the right hemisphere saw only that. He was then asked to choose from an array of pictures placed in full view in front of him. From the array of pictures, the shovel was chosen with the left hand and the chicken with the right. When asked why he chose these items, his left hemisphere speech center replied, 'Oh, that's simple. The chicken claw goes with the chicken, and you need a shovel to clean out the chicken shed.' Here the left brain, observing the left hand's response without knowing why it has picked that item, had to explain it. It will not say, 'I don't know.' Instead it interprets that response in a context consistent with what it knows, and all it knows is: chicken claw. It knows nothing about the snow scene, but it has to explain pointing to the shovel with the left hand. It has to find reasons for the behavior. We called this left hemisphere process the interpreter.' [M. Gazzaniga, Human, pg 294]

> 'These findings suggest that the interpretive mechanism of the left hemisphere is always hard at work, seeking the meaning of events. It is constantly looking for order and reason, even when there is none — which leads it continually to make mistakes. It tends to overgeneralize, frequently constructing a potential past as opposed to a true one.' [Gazzaniga, 'The Split Brain Revisited' in Scientific American July 1998, pg 54]

The interpretive function is not limited to visual perception. Experiments have revealed that memories and moods encoded in the split right brain are also subject to left brain interpretation. One can think of this as a higher level version of the perceptual filling-in of blind spots, body images, and phantom limbs one finds in stroke patients and amputees. Our minds don't like gaps and voids so it learns to cover them up.

Both hemispheres have a tendency to extract patterns from lower level input. As we saw earlier, the right brain specializes in the detection of low frequency spatial and acoustic groupings. The left brain is not so good at this sort of gestalt processing. But it far exceeds its counterpart in two other domains. The first is language. The second is the interpretive function. Given the uniqueness of human left brain capabilities and the commonality of gestalt perception in the animal kingdom, it seems likely that the right brain's superiority in global coherence is more a reflection of a loss of this function in the left brain than a gain of it in the right.

It appears that sometime in the evolution of the human animal, there arose a series of genetic mutations whose expression led to the development of neural architecture enabling rapid and flexible manipulation of activity patterns with symbolic meaning. One such system was syntax, which in turn gave rise to language. That was useful. Others included high level representations of body image, personality traits, and semantic and episodic memory. Those individuals with brains capable of juggling these representations with ease enjoyed reproductive and survival advantages compared to those who were not sufficiently 'with it.' The interpreter was born.

Just as the right brain, perhaps by default, can't help but see the world as silent, fleeting impressions confined to the here and now, the left brain experiences it as nuanced expressions firmly embedded in the extended space-time of one's identity. The highly integrated and yet differentiated richness and thickness of being one self come with the construction of an autobiographical narrative. The more frequently this narrative is edited, the more tempted one is to embellish it with false memories and poetic license, which, ironically, further serve to strengthen the illusion of self.

*****

The picture that is emerging is that the three different species of consciousness are distinct and potentially dissociable. *P consciousness*, with its irrevocable qualia, comes from the spotlight of attention. *S consciousness*, with its self-reflective ego, requires the machinery of P consciousness plus the left-brain interpreter. *A consciousness*, which depends on language, utilizes the left hemisphere language areas. All of these activated cortical areas are in close reciprocal contact with the thalamus. Inside each of us, there are multiple little Cartesian Theaters, each with its own separate modules and special access to the thalamus. All of these specialized circuits are continuously projecting multiple drafts of one's ongoing conscious life.

Just like a television broadcast of the Olympic games where multiple cameras in various locations simultaneously film different aspects of the subject, but the producers actively shift and edit from one view to another for the sake of the viewer at home, so it is with consciousness. Attention, biased both from top and bottom, is the producer that chooses which theater will broadcast the conscious experience. If attention's spotlight happens to shine on the temporal lobe, we become aware of the raw, elemental quality of objects and situations. If it shines on the parietal lobe, we become aware of our embodied physical self. If it shines on the left frontal lobe, we are able to articulate feelings into words and speech. Through it all, there emerges a sense of autobiographical unity: a metaconjunction of sorts, not of features in a visual setting, but of the composite aspects that make up one's identity. Antonio Damasio writes about this in his book, Descartes' Error:

'...In using the notion of self, I am in no way suggesting that *all* the contents of our minds are inspected by a single central knower and owner, and even less that such an entity would reside in a single brain place. I am saying, though, that our experiences tend to have a consistent perspective, as if there were indeed an owner and knower for most, though not all, contents. I imagine this perspective to be rooted in a relatively stable, endlessly repeated biological state. The source of the stability is the predominantly invariant structure and operation of the organism, and the slowly evolving elements of autobiographical data.' (A. Damasio, Descartes' Error, pg. 238)

'At each moment the state of self is constructed, from the ground up. It is an evanescent reference state, so continuously and consistently reconstructed that the owner never knows it is being remade unless something goes wrong with the remaking. The background feeling now, or the feeling of an emotion now, along with the non-body sensory signals now, happen to the concept of self as instantiated in the coordinate activity of multiple brain regions. But our self, or better even, our metaself, only 'learns' about that 'now' an instant later...Present continuously becomes past, and by the time we take stock of it we are in another present, consumed with planning the future, which we do on the stepping-stones of the past. The present is never here. We are hopelessly late for consciousness.' (pg. 240)

*****

The virtual reality of our conscious lives is an illusion. It is a phenomenon constructed by our neural machinery and then interpreted by our left hemisphere. It is altogether distinct from the reality of the physical world that really is out there. To appreciate an illusion for what it is, one must have access to a reality of a higher definition with which to contrast it. For instance, we know that our dreams, no matter how vivid, are just dreams when we compare them to the much richer experience of our waking lives. But the problem with the illusion of our waking lives is that this is the highest quality reality to which our brains have access. Consciousness is a wickedly clever adaptation for a life as a human animal; but for scientific inquiry, it veils the mind's eye from a clearer view.

Chapter 2

Decision Making

We feel sorry because we cry, angry because we strike, afraid because we tremble and not that we cry, strike or tremble because we are sorry, angry or fearful as the case may be.

William James
Principles of Psychology

Reason is, and ought only to be, the slave of the passions.

David Hume
Treatise of Human Nature

'Have you decided?' asked the attractive young woman at the adventure sports booth as she caught me glancing furtively at her. I'd always thought I wanted to go skydiving over the Swiss Alps. It would be the chance of a lifetime, a memory I would savor for years, an opportunity not to be missed. Strangely, now that the time had come, so did the doubts. I weighed the pros and cons. First, the cost: did I really want to pay two hundred dollars for a forty five second free fall? It had already been a pretty expensive vacation, and I would need some extra cash when I get to Paris. Next, the risk: what if I get sick or even killed? Should I stay or should I go? Then I had to decide which outfit to go with. Should I pick the company recommended in the guidebook as the one with the 'highest satisfaction rating', or a more obscure rival that listed a cheaper price? With all these things on my mind, I hesitated and walked over to the food stall. After the bratwurst and beer, I was more indecisive then ever. The woman was still there, smiling at me enticingly as if she had read my mind. Something clicked. 'Uh, can I sign up for one of your skydiving trips?' I asked her without thinking.

The small twin-engine plane was flying high over the Berner Oberland. To the left was the town of Interlaken flanked by its twin lakes. Just ahead were the snow-capped peaks of the Jungfrau massif rising majestically four thousand meters over the Swiss countryside. I was strapped snugly on to my skydiving instructor, Klaus, who was joking with a couple of Canadian girls making their first solo jumps. I tried to act relaxed too, knowing that this guy was an experienced professional with hundreds if not thousands of dives behind him. He was the one doing the work; all I had to do was enjoy the view. But I couldn't suppress my nerves. My throat was dry, my pulse raced, and my stomach was doing some strange churning, all beyond my control. Thoughts of doom kept rising to the surface. I recalled an incident in the local news a few years before about a diver whose parachute failed to open. What if something happened to Klaus? But I'd be a fool not to jump. I took the plunge.

The Dual System Architecture of Action

What comes to your mind when I ask you what you did today? You might say, 'oh, the usual; I drove to work, saw some clients, went to a staff presentation, came home and helped the kids with their homework.' But that's not what I mean. What did you really do? Well, now you might say, 'I shut off that damn alarm clock after hitting the snooze button four or five times, got out of bed, dragged a comb across my head, made my way downstairs and had a cup, looking up I noticed I was late, got dressed, started the car, drove to work... ' You can break it down even further: 'I inserted the key into the ignition, rotated my right wrist forwards until I heard the engine catch, released my hand, moved it towards the automatic gearshift, depressed the shift lock with my right thumb, pulled my forearm back while simultaneously plantar flexing my right foot onto the brake pedal and rotating my left shoulder to position my elbow above the driver's side lock, which I then depressed by quickly adducting my arm, reached down between my legs and eased the seat back... '

The mundane activities of our daily lives that we recall and describe so casually are in fact abstractions made up of dozens and even thousands of discrete sequential action components that have nothing to do with one another except that they are lumped into composites to which we arbitrarily assign purpose. At the fundamental level, bunches of simple neuro-muscular contractions get the individual to do something (get out of bed, drag a comb across his head). This collective activity is given a label in our minds and becomes part of a greater goal (getting ready for work). The conscious interpreter continually monitors ongoing motor behavior with the purpose of guiding it to a specific endpoint. It assumes that everything we do has a purpose. But what can we say about the action before its interpretation?

Almost everything we do lies beneath the surface of consciousness. We are not aware of every footstep or eye blink we make, nor would we want to be. There are more important things to think about. Most situations can be handled relatively well with pre-prepared responses. Like all organisms, humans thrive on regularity. Our environments are predictable. The sun always rises in the east, Friday afternoon is a time we look forward to, we always have to pay our mortgages at the beginning of each month. We are creatures of habit that take the same route to the supermarket, store the pots and pans on the same shelves, and bathe ourselves the same way day after day, week after week. These behaviors become so repetitive that it would be wasteful of mental resources to pay special attention to them. So we have evolved not to.

Psychologists have long noted that there seem to be two distinct systems of cognition at work in the human brain. An automatic system which neuroscientists call *system one* allows us to navigate our world and do things that are routine and not complex, such as eating or brushing our teeth. The automatic system is housed in the brainstem, midbrain, and limbic regions below the cerebral cortex, areas that evolved in our fish-like ancestors hundreds of millions of years ago. Over all this time, it has been crafted to be especially fast, efficient, and effortless. For the vast majority of animal species, the entire brain operates on system one.

In humans, there is a second system that came online several million years ago. *System two* is slower, clumsier, and takes a lot more work to get going. But it can solve more complicated problems in much more creative ways. Its neural correlates reside throughout the cerebral cortex, where they are illuminated by the attentional spotlight. Unlike the automatic system, its contents and processes are under conscious control. The great breakthrough of system two is its ability to 'reflect' back on itself, using those cortical loops I discussed in the last chapter. Instead of simply reacting to the world through the instantaneous deployment of pre-programmed motor schemas, this reflective system is able to perceive its own actions a split second after the fact. And as the loops go round and round the cylindrical stream of consciousness, the mind becomes more and more aware of its own awareness in a kind of metacognition. Simply put, the system two interface allows its users to know what they're doing. And why is it so important to know what you're up to? Because now you can be flexible; you have the option of modifying or inhibiting pre-programmed responses. And if you hook up the reflective system to the memory systems of the brain, whole new worlds of imagined possibilities open up.

In the complex world humans have created for themselves, the two systems complement each other and are best used together. We see system two in action when we drive around in a new city, converse with a blind date, or sweat through a job interview. These are activities that have a high degree of novelty, uncertainty, and unpredictability. No one expects to do a good job on autopilot. It takes conscious effort, concentration, and attention to tackle these situations.

The Elusive Search for Reason

Post-Freudian psychologists like to use the iceberg analogy when explaining the gap between conscious and automatic processing in the mind. Awareness is the brilliantly dazzling part of the iceberg we can see from the ship, while the unconscious is that dark menacing mass under the surface. Similarly, philosophers and mystics from Plato's time on have distinguished man's noble ability to reason from his animalistic passions. We see this dichotomy in the arts in the contrast between Classicism and Romanticism. We see it in politics in the tension between idealists who believe in man's perfectibility and cynics who believe we are naturally flawed. Writers from Shakespeare to Steinbeck have used this motif as the basis for many of the classics of literature. It certainly makes compelling drama. Man is confronted by a moral dilemma. He is tempted by his emotions (lust, greed, jealousy, pride), and in a moment of weakness, he gives in. But in the end, he sees the light of reason, and does the right thing, saving himself, and the story, in the process. The epic age-old struggle between reason and passion is a central theme in religion and jurisprudence and has been stylized into art, architecture, music, and poetry. Even science has not been immune. Until quite recently, most psychologists ascribed to the Freudian notion that humans are constantly struggling with subconscious passions that interfere with the decision making process. The implication is that we should make decisions in a dispassionate, rational way.

This conventional view of rationality and emotion has two fatal flaws. The first is the belief that because emotions are irrational, they must be bad. Emotions are simply physiological responses that happen to play a crucial role in many of the decisions we make every day. We will return to the role of emotions and feelings later in this chapter. The second flaw is the idea that there is a part of the human mind that is purely rational. Let's tackle this myth first.

Try this: are there more words in the English language starting with the letter **r** or with **r** in the third position? What are the odds that an American will die next year in a tornado, an airline crash, an attack of asthma, or accidental drowning? Did more people die of homicide or suicide last year? Most people give the same answers to these simple questions. Surprisingly, most people are consistently wrong. In fact, there are many more words with **r** in the third place (*hurt, farm, bird, car, curious, tireless, worried*) than in the first (*red, ride, read, road, raid*). But it is easy to think of a word beginning with a certain letter; all we have to do is pronounce the sound and the words just pop up automatically. We can't use this trick so well when the sound isn't in front. Similarly, all of us who watch cable news on a regular basis are endlessly exposed to sensational stories of murder, mayhem, and all manner of disasters natural and man-made. Suicides, drownings, and asthma fatalities don't make the headlines, because they are so common. So they don't come to mind when we're asked to think about their relative frequency. As rational people, we may understand that ease of recall is not a good indicator of frequency. But that's not how our brains work. In the 1970's, the Israeli psychologists Danny Kahneman and Amos Tversky discovered that when making judgments under uncertain conditions, people consistently deploy certain *heuristics*, or biases. One of them is the *availability heuristic*, illustrated by the examples above. When we have to make a judgment about the frequency or likelihood of something where the actual statistics are not available to us, we make an educated guess based on what is available to our mind at the time.

Here's another experiment dreamed up by Kahneman and Tversky. Take Linda, a hypothetical 31 year-old, single, vegetarian, well-educated woman. She was active in student politics back in college, and participated in anti-nuclear demonstrations. Subjects were asked to rank, in order of probability, various possible outcomes in Linda's future, including 'bank teller', and 'bank teller active in the feminist movement.' Most subjects reported that Linda would more likely become a feminist bank teller than simply a bank teller. But this is impossible, as the set of 'feminist bank tellers' is a subset of 'bank tellers', feminist or otherwise. This is an example of the *representativeness heuristic*. Given our stereotypes, Linda is more representative of a feminist bank teller than a non-feminist one. Never mind that this isn't the question we're asked: it is the answer that comes automatically because it fits the pattern we have already created subconsciously. The mind handles images and examples better than abstractions and statistics. Just think back to your college days sweating over your probability and statistics finals. Representativeness is also at play in experiments where people were found to be willing to donate more money to *one* orphan in Africa (whose picture and profile are seen on TV) than to an aid agency that funds food programs and education for thousands of African orphans. A single visual representative is worth more than a large number on paper. Advertisers have known about this for a long time, and have put it to good use, for example, in commercials for environmental protection that pull at our heartstrings by featuring a weeping Native American man or a starving polar bear cub jumping off a melting ice floe after his mother.

A third rule of thumb our minds use in making judgments is called *anchoring*. Consider this experiment: write down the last three digits of your phone number. Now answer this historical question: in what year did the Western Roman Empire collapse? Psychologists found that subjects with relatively high phone numbers guessed a higher year (sometimes hundreds of years greater) than those with lower phone numbers. In another experiment, subjects were shown a set of lines before being asked to guess the length of the Mississippi River. Those who were primed with relatively short lines tended to grossly underestimate the actual length while those shown longer lines tended to overshoot the mark. Strikingly, the estimates often differed by an order of magnitude. What does one's phone number have to do with the collapse of the Roman Empire (476 AD)? What does the length of lines on a piece of paper have to do with the Mississippi River? Nothing, other than serving as psychological 'anchors' from which blind guesses are launched. What these experiments tell us, apart from the fact that Americans are woefully ignorant of history and geography, is that all sorts of random stimuli can act as anchors. People use anchors to make judgments all the time. Shoppers for a used car often fixate on the odometer, ignoring all the rest; a fellow going out on a blind date may concentrate on his partner's crooked tooth, instead of her personality. Often, these biases serve as accurate fitness indicators that reveal something of the underlying quality of the product, and our minds have evolved to use them. But sometimes we latch onto anchors that have nothing to do with the subject at hand, causing us to make erroneous judgments.

Anchoring, availability, and representativeness are cognitive biases that serve as short cuts in the conscious decision making process. They are rough-edged empiric rules of thumb that served our ancestors well in the days when making an accurate split-second decision literally meant the difference between the chance to mate and pass on one's genes or becoming someone else's dinner. Creative experiments in the psych lab have revealed these heuristics to be neither precise nor rational, but in the real world they are often effective.

Under the Surface

Left to its own devices, system two is governed by rules of thumb. We, or at least the interpreter in our left hemisphere, like to think that reason is the guiding light that shapes our judgments and decisions, but that usually isn't the case. The outside world influences our choices and judgments through its anchors, representatives, and availabilities. We justify them as rational after the fact. Our consciousness is also warped by subconscious factors constantly welling up to the surface. In a series of elegant experiments, the psychologist John Bargh discovered that our behavior can be dictated by subliminal influences as much as by conscious intent. One example involves subjects who were made to sit in front of a computer screen and do a spatial recognition task (the decoy experiment), while certain key words like 'Florida' and 'wrinkles' were flashed on the screen for a few milliseconds. When the subjects were asked to walk down the hall afterwards, they walked more slowly after they had been primed by words that suggested old age and infirmity than after words that did not. The subjects hadn't had time to recognize the words on the screen, and were unaware that the speed of their walk was being measured. These experiments and their variants have been replicated repeatedly, leaving no doubt as to the existence of the subconscious priming effect.

Environmental factors as trivial as background color can also prime the cognitive machinery. In a recent experiment, Professor Juliet Zhu at the University of British Columbia found that volunteers performed better on computerized tests of verbal recall and visual attention when the background screen color was red, while they tended to do better on tests of creativity (coming up with different uses for a brick) when done against a blue background. Another study found that athletes who wore red in boxing, wrestling, and tae kwon do at the 2004 Olympic games won 60% of their matches against opponents who wore blue. It appears that longer wavelengths of light subliminally signal danger (fire or blood, for instance), alerting the cognitive machinery to focus on whatever task is at hand. Colors associated with shorter wavelengths signal serenity and tranquility (the sea and the sky) and have a calming effect on consciousness. Cool colors are not as conducive to focused attention, but may enhance creative thought and the ability to see the big picture.

Cognitive psychologists have begun to recognize the remarkably widespread phenomenon of *embodied cognition,* the notion that mental processes are grounded in the physical body and its interactions with the outside world. In a recent study, researchers at Yale University divided a pool of subjects into two groups. The first group was instructed to hold a cup of hot coffee for a few minutes while reading a passage about a fictional character. The second group was told to do this while holding a cup of iced coffee. When asked afterwards, the subjects with the hot beverage tended to describe the character as 'warmer' when compared with those who had been holding the iced coffee. The psychologist Nils Jostmann of the University of Amsterdam discovered that subjects who had been holding a heavy clipboard during a test session were more likely to estimate an unfamiliar currency as having a higher value when compared with those who had been holding a lighter clipboard. These fascinating experiments suggest that our social and economic judgments are often subtly influenced by totally unrelated sensory perceptions. This also works in reverse: simple perceptions can be biased by our conscious judgments. In another series of experiments, Professor Jostmann's group found that students who were told that a particular book was vital to their coursework judged that book to be heavier than did the students who were not told this. Psychologists at the University of Toronto found that subjects who were instructed to recall an incident in which they were rejected by their peers judged the ambient temperature of the room they were in to be lower than subjects who were asked to recall a neutral incident.

What is clear from these studies is that there are multiple routes leading to behavior, and most of them are subconscious. We tend to overemphasize the 'willfully-driven freeway' in the decision making process. We believe that we do what we do simply because we want to do it. What we don't realize is that environmental context, such as the color of the background or the temperature of our fingers, can dramatically influence goal-directed behavior. These factors constantly and automatically ignite associated motor programs. It seems to me that we expend more willful effort trying to rein in our subconscious demons than in actually initiating behavior. In this respect, we are unlike all other species of life on earth. System one is all they have, and all they need; consciousness is not included in the start up kit. Human consciousness is a 100,000 year-old evolutionary add-on that is really more of a luxury than a necessity.

The discovery of the unconscious and its guiding role in our lives dates back many centuries before Freud. Greek, Buddhist, and Hindu mystics in pre-Christian times knew about it. But until recently, this notion has not had much impact on those studying the human decision making process. Things have changed. Spurred on by breakthroughs in brain imaging and neurochemistry over the last several decades, cognitive psychologists and behavioral economists are incorporating the workings of the unconscious mind into more established theories of decision making to create a brand new field called *neuro-economics*.

Neuroeconomists started by challenging an axiom invented by an eighteenth century Dutch mathematician named Daniel Bernoulli to describe the expected behavior of a 'rational agent' when confronted with a financial decision. Bernoulli believed that any free and reasonable person would choose a particular course of action if the resulting chance of gain and the value of that gain outweighs the value of not so choosing: Expected Value (of a choice)= Odds of Gain x Value of Gain. For instance, it would make sense to purchase a $1000 insurance policy to protect the shipment of $100,000 worth of property (a 1% sure cost) if the estimated risk of total loss were, say, 2%. The job of the classical economist is the rather straightforward task of calculating these odds and values. Fair enough, except that much of the time, people don't make the decisions the economists predict they would. There are two main reasons for this. The first is that their brains follow those quick and dirty rules of thumb I mentioned earlier. Heuristics of availability, representativeness, and anchoring cloud our ability to calculate the odds accurately. The second reason is that there are serious built-in limitations on our ability to perceive the value of a future gain.

Are We Happy Yet?

All animals are motivated to behave in ways that maximize their chance to survive and reproduce. Thanks to Charles Darwin, we now know that such behavior is inherited and selected, spreading through populations and adapting to habitats far and wide. And thanks to developmental neuroscientists, we also know that most such behavior is preprogrammed into animal brains via genes that make nerve cells work together in wondrous ways. In every animal, goal-directed behavior is automatic and unconscious, driven by a combination of external stimuli and internal physiology; it is fast, effortless, and, for most intents and purposes, accurate. So, too, is the human animal prone to all sorts of automatic behavior prompted by subliminal suggestion. But humans still cling to the arrogant belief that they are somehow qualitatively different from, even superior to, all other animals. Is this so, or has science finally stripped us of our last shred of self-righteous vanity, revealing us to be nothing more than a scrawny naked ape with a freakishly swollen forehead?

Rest assured that we are different in many important ways from even our closest surviving relatives, the chimpanzees and bonobos of Africa. Perhaps the most significant difference is our ability to forecast and plan for the distant future. Simple animals like fruit flies can learn a few things through conditioning, such as associating a smell with a noxious stimulus. Birds and monarch butterflies undertake epic migrations of thousands of miles. Apes and dolphins can fashion crude tools to grab inaccessible food items. The first is an example of an unconscious conditioned reflex. The second is a genetically encoded neural program. Only the last case can truly be considered a consciously willed goal-directed behavior. But even those actions are completely driven by the here and now. The chimp inserts the straw into the termite nest *right here* because it wants to eat those termites *right now*. What makes humans unique is our propensity to consciously and compulsively engage in complex long-range planning. I plan to go online to order study material for my medical board exam so that I can be ready when I take it next year. We work hard and save money to invest so that we can pay for our children's education 18 years from now. We do these things to reach distant goals that we believe are valuable.

The human brain has a wonderful tool for complex planning called *working memory*. It allows me to hold a small amount of information on-line (such as the phone number for the nearest pharmacy) while I manipulate other unrelated information (the dosage of Gertrude's thyroid medication) necessary for a larger task (making sure Gertrude gets her pills before she goes off on her Mediterranean cruise). Working memory is part of a larger domain of cognition called *executive function*. We will explore the neuroanatomy of executive function and dysfunction later. But now back to values and goals.

What makes something valuable to us? Why do we set goals and strive for them? How do we feel when we achieve them? The simple answer is that we like things that make us happy, so we try to maximize our happiness. On second thought, this isn't always the case. There are many things that we might consider valuable or worthwhile which do not necessarily make us happy (waiting in line at the supermarket, working in the office all night, wearing a condom, jumping on a live hand grenade). But all of them are choices that we make with the expectation of future utility, however remote. Cutting the line means that you might be caught and chastised. Not working all night means missing the deadline and possibly forfeiting a promotion. Not wearing a condom means that she might get pregnant or that you might end up with AIDS. Not jumping on the grenade might mean death to your buddies and life-long survivor's guilt. All the conscious actions we take, all the choices we make are done with the intention of achieving happiness.

What is happiness and what is its utility? Strictly defined, happiness is a neuro-physiological state characterized by the release of serotonin and dopamine throughout the central nervous system. It is a signal to and within the brain that inhibits further goal seeking behavior for the moment. Its adaptive function in creating a homeostatic environment is unmistakable. In this general sense, one could say that many species of animals experience happiness of some sort, but not in the rich nuanced way that we can. Thanks to our large cerebral cortex, with its working memory, cortical-thalamic loops, and the left hemisphere interpreter, humans are uniquely able to experience extra dimensions of happiness, recall happy moments from the past and play them out in sequence, and imagine being happy now or in some future time. Creating pleasant moments in our minds helps us to plan a means of achieving them in reality. But just as we saw with judgment under uncertainty, the problem with affective forecasting is that it is subject to systematic biases.

Affective Misforecasting

Happiness is a fleeting sensation that need not even enter awareness. It is easy to measure: just ask someone how happy they are right now, say, on a scale of one to ten. Unless the subject is deliberately lying to you, the answer is more accurate than anything you can gauge from a fancy brain scan. People usually don't have delusions about their current feelings. The problems come when they are asked to remember how happy they were in the past, or worse, to predict how happy they may feel in the future.

Despite its many quirks, perception is much more accurate than either memory or imagination. And the most veridical perceptions are those furthest down on the neural pathway. Just as the images sensed by our retinal cells are progressively edited as they get processed in the visual cortex, the emotions felt through our amygdala are progressively edited as they get processed in the prefrontal cortex. The final copies of both the images and the feelings that arrive in our extended consciousness are no longer pure. Consciousness contaminates the purity of sensation. Perhaps this is why many people report that some of their happiest moments are spent doing mindlessly repetitive behaviors that they have mastered, such as dancing, crocheting, or playing basketball. The psychologist Mihaly Csikszentmihalyi describes a phenomenon he calls *flow*, the positive feeling gained by engaging in a well learned task that is neither so easy as to become boring, nor so difficult that it requires much conscious effort. Athletes describe this as being 'in the zone'.

It's remarkable how prone we are to misjudging our future feelings. Just think of the last time you went food shopping on an empty stomach. Did you end up eating all the junk you bought? Or how about when you joined the Megafitness Gym after the Christmas holidays. How often have you been working out? Or, to take a more serious example, how would you feel a year after losing your spouse? Most would say that they would be devastated and depressed. But studies have shown that people generally rebound quite well a year after the death of a loved one. These examples reveal the systematic errors we make in predicting the future. Because our awareness of the present is so much more compelling and detailed than images of a possible future, predictions of the future are inevitably anchored in perceptions of the present. The psychologist Daniel Gilbert puts this eloquently in his book <u>Stumbling on Happiness</u>:

> 'If the past is a wall with some holes, the future is a hole with no walls. Memory *uses* the filling-in trick, but imagination *is* the filling-in trick, and if the present lightly colors our remembered pasts, it thoroughly infuses our imagined futures.
>
> …Because time is such a slippery concept, we tend to imagine the future as the present with a twist, thus our imagined tomorrows inevitably look like slightly twisted versions of today. The reality of the moment is so palpable and powerful that it holds imagination in a tight orbit from which it never fully escapes.' [<u>Stumbling on Happiness</u> p126, 162]

We humans have a wonderful tool that prepares us for the future, our working memory/executive function system built into our prefrontal cortex. But too often its ingenuity is based on incorrect predictions of the future that are anchored to our perceptions of the present. Our memories of past experiences are also subject to misinterpretation. One such culprit is *recency bias*, discovered by Danny Kahneman in the 1980's. He conducted a series of experiments involving volunteers dipping their hands into icy cold water. Pretty painful stuff. Remarkably, volunteers found that it was more painful to endure this temperature for a minute than to follow the same minute in ice water with thirty seconds in a slightly warmer bath. This doesn't make sense unless we realize that our minds are responding not to the sum total of painful moments, but rather to the most recent painful moment (which was less intense in the latter session). Additionally, when we recollect our past experiences, the handful of extreme moments are much more salient, and thus better remembered, than the many average moments.

Frames and References

Try this thought experiment: there is an epidemic in your country. If you take no action, 600 people will die. There are two possible treatments. Under treatment A, 200 of those people will surely die. With treatment B, there is a 2/3 chance that no one will die, but a 1/3 chance that all 600 will die. As the health minister of this country, you must now decide which treatment to administer. If you're like most people, you would choose treatment B, because it offers the chance of saving everyone.

Now let's frame the scenario differently. Again, you're faced with an epidemic that will kill 600 people. Treatment A definitely saves 400 of them. Treatment B offers a 2/3 chance of saving all 600, but a 1/3 chance of saving no one. In this situation, it turns out that most people would now go with treatment A, because a sure thing is better than a risk when it comes to saving lives. Now read the two cases over again carefully. The odds of survival for each treatment are identical in both formulations; the only thing different is the wording. And, yet, context matters.

When a choice is framed as a loss (200 people will die), we are much more averse to choosing it than when it is framed as a gain (400 people will be saved), even though the odds are the same. This is known as *loss aversion bias*, yet another of Kahneman and Tversky's many discoveries. The sting of losing is so much more painful than the joy of winning is pleasurable that we fool ourselves into valuing something that we possess more than something that we don't. This makes sense in evolutionary terms when we remember that our ancestors frequently risked losing their lives, in exchange for just another opportunity for feeding or fucking. Take your pick.

The following curve depicts how loss aversion works. As most of us are aware, our subjective experience of happiness or value doesn't follow a linear relationship with net gains. On the right side of the graph, we can see that if we have very little to start with, even a small gain feels big. But if we already have a lot, than it will take much more to make us feel richer. This is the familiar law of diminishing returns. Now look at the left side of the graph. When we deal with losses, the same sort of relationship we encounter with gains occurs in reverse. Any reduction from baseline is painful, but if we keep losing more, the accrued pain is proportionally adulterated. But the interesting discovery is that the *slope* of the curve on the right is much greater than that of the curve on the left. The intensity of the pain of loss is greater than the intensity of the pleasure of a comparable gain.

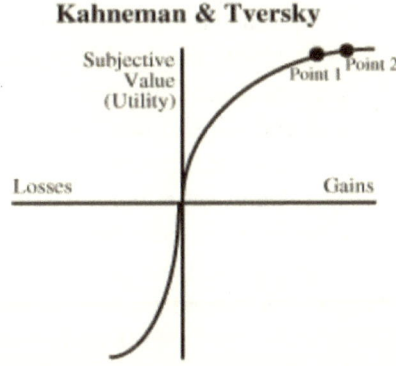

Figure 8: loss aversion

Now let's move on to the link between wealth and happiness. We all know that money can't always buy happiness. But it is an important component of happiness, otherwise why would people invest so much time and toil to get it? Economists since the time of Bernoulli knew the logarithmic relationship between wealth and utility [see the right side of figure 1]. The more wealth one has, the less utility or happiness one gets for a further increase in wealth. In other words, there is a big difference between not having enough and having enough, but not much difference between having enough and having more than your fair share. The problem is knowing when to say enough is enough.

As we saw in the last chapter, the human mind is sensitive not to absolute values, but rather to relative changes in value. Neurons in the visual cortex respond to contrast rather than to absolute brightness, for example. This is as true for affective judgment as it is for visual perception. The multi-millionaire surrounded by billionaires will feel poorer than the guy in the working class neighborhood with a half-million dollar mini-mansion. Similarly, one's present wealth is evaluated in the context of one's past and future wealth. Of two people who both currently have a million dollars, the one who just lost $100,000 in the stock market will feel poorer than the one who just scored a profit of $100,000. A job promising a $50,000 salary this year and $75,000 next year is more attractive than one offering $75,000 this year and $50,000 next year. What has been so often said of life is also true of wealth: what counts is the journey, not the destination.

On a cold January morning in 2009 in the small German town of Blaubeuren, Adolph Merckle deliberately jumped in front of a speeding locomotive. At the time of his death, Herr Merckle had a net worth in excess of nine billion U.S. dollars, making him one of the hundred richest people in the world. At 74, he still enjoyed good health and the company of his loving wife and children. Yet this highly regarded businessman had been driven to desperation. In the preceding year, his investment company was caught in the throes of a global financial meltdown. Hoping to shore up mounting losses, Merckle made a bold gamble by speculating billions of euros on a bet that the ailing Volkswagen Company's shares would fall. It proved to be a miscalculation that cost him 500 million euros. Rather than dealing with the guilt and shame of defaulting on his bank loans, Merckle took his own life.

This sort of behavior would seem extreme to most. How many of us would kill to have Merckle's wealth rather than die in spite of it? But then we were not in his shoes. Merckle's actions become clearer when one considers how his losses must have felt for someone accustomed to great profits and success. He was still immensely wealthy, but in the end, it was relative loss that mattered. There is truth to the adage, 'the higher you climb, the further you fall'. He still had his family and his health, but his outlook on the future was firmly anchored to the magnitude and suddenness of his loss. Loss aversion, recency bias, and the anchoring heuristic all conspired in producing Merckle's myopia for the future.

Dopamine's Drive

The key to decision-making is the neurotransmitter, *dopamine*. It is the biochemical signal that primes our brains to recognize goals and rewards, and confers value onto our actions, from the most automatic and mundane, like walking and eating, to the fantastically difficult and unusual, such as climbing mountains and writing books. Without our dopamine neurons, we would literally die of starvation.

What's so important about dopamine? Long before humans could talk and make conscious decisions, long before humans or any other primates even evolved, more humble creatures were making crucial life and death decisions. Worms and insects had to recognize food, find mates, and flee predators. Much of this behavior was and still is controlled by automatic circuits or reflexes triggered by stimuli. Our distant ancestors soon evolved genetic mechanisms coding for the necessary neural hardware. But genes can only define brains at a coarse level. You are born with a fixed set of DNA sequences, and the range of gene expression, although remarkable, is neither fast nor flexible enough to allow you and your brain to go shopping, cook dinner, or play the stock market.

Life is unpredictable. The supermarket may be closed, your car may have just had a flat, Citygroup stocks may be at an all time low. There are no genetic programs for dealing with stuff like that. You have to make conscious decisions based on evidence, options, and predictions, mixed with gut feelings. All of this is done by dopamine neurons. This remarkable organic compound is the common thread that ties motion, emotion, and cognition together.

But first some neurochemistry. Dopamine is synthesized at the axon terminal from the essential amino acid, *tyrosine*, by two enzymes, *tyrosine hydroxylase* and *DOPA decarboxylase*. The first enzyme, which converts tyrosine into the dopamine precursor, *L-DOPA*, is the rate-limiting step. L-DOPA or *levodopa* (commonly packaged as the drug *sinemet*) is the most widely used treatment for Parkinson's disease, a disorder associated with the destruction of dopaminergic neurons in the basal ganglia. Once synthesized, dopamine is stored in vesicles near the synaptic junction. Stimulation of the dopamine neuron will cause the vesicles to fuse with the axon membrane, releasing the neurotransmitter into the cleft where it can bind to and activate any of five different dopamine receptors on the target cell. Dopamine receptors are large molecules that span the post-synaptic membrane (the dendritic surface of the receiving neuron) seven times, and relay the dopamine signal to other proteins and enzymes in the signal transduction pathway, eventually leading to changes in the function and sometimes the structure of the synapse. In addition to triggering an action potential in the target cell, the dopamine signal may induce synaptic modifications such as the pruning of connections or even the sprouting of new dendrites. These changes may be transient (a few seconds), or long lasting (years or a lifetime).

Once its work at the synapse is done, the dopamine is removed from the cleft by a transporter protein on the presynaptic membrane, returned to the axon from which it originated, and either broken down by an enzyme called *monoamine oxidase* (MAO) or repackaged into vesicles where it can later be reused. Another class of pharmaceuticals somewhat useful for the early stages of Parkinson's disease is designed to inhibit monoamine oxidase. These *MAO inhibitors* (such as *selegiline* and *cogentin*) prevent the degradation of dopamine, allowing more of it to act where needed.

And now, some neuroanatomy. Most of the brain's dopamine neurons are found in the *substantia nigra* and ventral tegmental areas of the midbrain, and there is a minor cluster in the hypothalamus. From these regions, their axons project to many other parts of the brain. There are four distinct dopamine projection systems. The *tuberoinfundibular system* regulates prolactin secretion. This endocrine component of dopamine is not related to the realm of decision-making, and will not go into it. The other three systems are more relevant. The *nigrostriatial system* courses from the substantia nigra to the *striatum* (the putamen and the caudate nuclei). The *mesolimbic system* extends from the ventral tegmentum to the limbic structures (the nucleus accumbens, entorhinal cortex, and the amygdala) as well as to the hippocampus. Finally, the *mesocortical system* connects the ventral tegmentum with the cortex, especially the prefrontal and anterior cingulate regions.

Too little dopamine in the substantia nigra causes movement disorders such as Parkinson's disease. But too much of it in axonal projections into the cortex can cause psychotic disorders such as schizophrenia. This is why drugs that block dopamine receptors are used as antipsychotics. This also explains why the treatments for Parkinson's disease can cause psychosis, and why antipsychotics, especially the higher potency ones like *prolixen* and *haldol*, often cause Parkinsonian-like side effects called *tardive diskinesia.*

Animals are preprogrammed to be attracted to certain appetitively salient stimuli. For instance, the sight of food, the warmth of shelter, or the attractive scent of a member of the opposite sex. They are also preprogrammed to withdraw from certain noxious stimuli, such as electric shocks and creatures with gaping mouths and sharp teeth. The perception of these stimuli activates preset sensory-motor loops which cause the animal to approach or flee as the case may warrant. Such behavior need not be conscious (and usually isn't). The activity of the motor component of the loop is automatically deployed whenever the sensory component is activated. However, a long or interrupted interval between the stimulus and the response is difficult for the brain to sustain. This is where the dopamine system comes into play.

Midbrain neurons that use dopamine as their neurotransmitter fire tonically at some basal rate. These cells are connected to and activated by other neurons in the sensory pathway. Dopamine neurons fire during the period between the perception of the appetitive stimulus and the realization of the goal, for example the smell of a warm meal and its taste on the tongue. The firing rate is sustained throughout the delay and tends to remain unaffected by distracters. Some believe that the greater the perceived value of the goal, the higher the firing rate. But this might be looking at the situation backwards. What's actually happening is that the higher firing rate *correlates* with greater value. Dopamine is therefore an *expectation signal* that tells the cortex there is something it needs to do. However, the dopamine neuron itself does not know what the goal is; its signal is a highly useful, if nondescript, motivational tag that reminds us that there is a decision to be made.

A perhaps even more important aspect of the dopamine system is its role in learning and memory. In the early years of the last century, the Russian physiologist Ivan Pavlov discovered the principles of conditioned learning. Dogs who normally salivate at the sight of food (the unconditioned stimulus) can be conditioned to salivate to the sound of a bell (the conditioned stimulus) after a few trials in which the bell coincides with food. This is a classic example of the dopamine system at work. A stimulus followed by an expected reward (the sight of food followed by the action of eating) activates the dopamine neuron slightly compared with baseline. But a stimulus followed by a novel or unexpected reward (the bell followed by the meal) makes the dopamine system fire away like mad. The neural ensemble representing the sound of the bell and that representing a belly full of food are linked together by the mesolimbic/mesocortical dopamine systems. New connections are forged, memories are planted, and the animal learns to associate the novel stimulus with the reward. The dopamine anticipation signal has been transferred. On the other hand, unexpected punishments, such as an electric shock following a bell, will depress the dopamine neuron's firing rate well below baseline. For this reason, the neuroscientist Wolfram Schultz of Cambridge University has called the dopamine neurons the 'retina of the reward system'.

Virtually all drugs of abuse from alcohol and nicotine to marijuana, amphetamine, ketamine, cocaine, and the opiates exert their effects by enhancing dopamine transmission in various ways, most commonly by blocking the *dopamine transporter molecule*. What makes these substances so addictive is that they produce near instantaneous dopamine surges several fold greater than in normal physiological circumstances. The resulting rush of pleasure and the feeling of reward are decoupled from external circumstances. No sound of a bell or sight of food is required; the dopamine rewards the brain without an anticipation signal. Drug abusers are motivated, of course. But their goal is simply getting their next hit. Given a steady supply of dope, the dopamine is its own reward, and all other appetitive stimuli, including the most primal urges of sex and food, pale in comparison. A happy addict would gladly spend his day in a self-absorbed haze, with nothing in the real world to arouse him.

On the other hand, there are people, who through no fault of their own, lie at the other end of the spectrum. Studies on identical twins raised in separate adoptive families have shown that risk-taking and novelty-seeking behavior seem to have a strong genetic component with a heritability rate around 40%. Molecular geneticists have linked some of this heritability to a mutation in the fourth dopamine receptor (*D4*). The more common form of D4 normally has a 48 base-pair region in one of its cytoplasmic domains. There is a less common variant of this gene in which this segment is repeated seven times. This longer form of the D4 receptor appears to be less effective in transducing the dopamine signal. Individuals who are homozygous (having two copies) for the longer D4 receptor were found to engage in more risk-taking behaviors (such as skydiving, motorcycle racing, gambling, and drug taking) than those in the general population. It may be that they get less of dopamine's motivational bang for the buck, and need to make up for it in other ways.

Interestingly, developmental biologists have found that fruit flies and nematode worms also seem to have variants in novelty seeking. The developmental biologist Cornelia Bargmann observed that in a given population of worms, some individuals will stay in one place and slowly feed on whatever bacteria (their favorite food) was around in the immediate vicinity, while others would forage all over sampling here and there. Professor Bargmann subsequently discovered that there was a gene responsible for this behavioral variation. This gene has a human homologue that may correlate with similar social behavior. It's easy to see how such genetic variants could have evolved. Conservative foraging strategies, whether for food, fortunes, or females, is generally safer, cheaper, and more reliable than taking wild chances. But as every compulsive gambler knows, life is a crapshoot that occasionally rewards the reckless risk-taker. It usually doesn't pay to take undue risks, so those with genes for conservative behavior are more likely to survive and populate the world with offspring who also have those genes. But sometimes it pays so much that those few with genes for risk-taking or novelty seeking are able to sire more than their fair share of offspring with similar personalities. We shall encounter this balance again in terms of liberals and conservatives in the last chapter.

Motivation for Motion

Decision-making in its most basic form implies physical action. The motor components of brains came on-line prior to the cognitive components. Our less advanced ancestors were acting in and reacting to their little worlds long before they evolved the capacity to internalize their thoughts. This is a natural history written in dopamine. But first let's review the neuroscience of motor control.

Imagine any voluntary activity: answering the phone, brushing your teeth, playing the piano, catching a football pass, grabbing a cold beer from the fridge, driving down a rain-slicked road at night. We think of them as single acts. They are not. Each is a complex composite made up of little movements like reaching, pulling, and twisting in a specific, finely-coordinated sequence. Each little movement is carried out by teams of muscles under the command of their corresponding motor nerves from the spinal cord. But voluntary movements are more than simply the sum of their parts. When we walk into the kitchen to get that beer, we experience a unitary and coherent action, rather than the dozens or hundreds of discrete hand, finger, and eye movements and thousands of muscle contractions that go into every successful act of beer retrieval. What we are conscious of is a high level action schema. Just as in sensory perception, where the mind's eye sees a holistic representation of the real world rather than thousands of disjointed little pixels, the motor system gives the brain an integrated representation of motor activity.

Voluntary acts share a common theme: incoming sensory perception linked to outgoing motor activity. They are rather like the classic knee-jerk reflex, but at a higher level of complexity. To a wide receiver in football, an incoming pass is much more than a spiraling two-dimensional oval in space. It becomes part of a 'play' involving the positions, trajectories, identities, and motives of the other players relative to the receiver, the field, the football, the time clock, and the score of the game. At this juncture, both perceptual and motor representations are abstract. Sensory perceptions are bound into something coherent: a creative facsimile of the real world. It is *on top of* this facsimile that voluntary motor plans are constructed.

Anatomically, the sensory-motor loop involves a linkage between the parts of the brain that contain high-order representations of sensory perception (the association areas of the sensory cortex) and the parts of the brain that contain high-order representations of motor preparation (the supplementary and premotor cortices, along with the cerebellum and the basal ganglia). Information in all of these regions is organized somatotopically. That is, each part of the body is mapped onto a corresponding part of the brain. Certain parts of the body, such as the face and fingers, receive much more attention in both the sensory and motor maps. This is why the sensory and motor *homunculi* are so funny looking. Evolutionarily, this makes sense. We use our fingers and mouths to interact with the world a lot more than, say, our backs. An individual who, for whatever genetic reason, had slightly more sensitive lips or slightly more dexterous fingers might have had a slightly better chance of getting a female to have sex with him. The genes that build brains with slightly better face and hand representation became more prevalent in the population, eventually resulting in the brains we all have today.

Somatotopic organization exists in the primary sensory and motor areas, their respective higher order cortices, and even in the cerebellum and the basal ganglia. The cerebellum, in fact, has three separate body maps. Activity in the higher-order motor cortex represents the earlier stages of action preparation, for example, generally thinking about walking into the kitchen. Activity in the primary motor strip, the cerebellum, and the basal ganglia represents the fine-tuning of actions in real-time, such as opening the refrigerator door or reaching for the bottle of Budweiser on the bottom shelf.

The sensory-motor arc is more than just a linkage of information stored in the sensory cortex with that stored in the motor cortex. There are two important structures beyond the cortex: the cerebellum and the basal ganglia, each of which make sensory-motor loops of their own. Let's briefly examine them.

The cerebellum is a dense package of neurons located in the back of the brain. It has its own cortex and subcortical nuclei, and its surface contains several body maps, rather like a miniature cerebral cortex. The cerebellum receives sensory input via the brainstem and has outputs to the motor system both directly to the spinal cord and indirectly via the thalamus and motor cortex. The cerebellum's unique feature is a dual input channel, which modulates incoming sensory activity. The first channel, called the *parallel fiber network*, receives raw input from the visual, auditory, vestibular, and motor systems in real time. The second channel, called the *climbing fiber network*, receives partially processed input representing the previous movement, with a slight delay. The parallel fiber network diffusely stimulates its particular area of the cerebellum (its receptive field), while the climbing fiber network strongly, but transiently, inhibits it. Thus input to the cerebellum from a particular part of the body arrives in two paths, producing an initial activation, followed by a delayed inhibition. This prevents a movement from being inappropriately prolonged, allowing a smooth transition to the next movement. The end result of cerebellar activity on motor output is an ongoing time correction signal. The motor response to sensory input via the parallel fibers is constantly modulated by feed-forward cerebellar activity via the climbing fibers. The cerebellum is essential for proper balance, coordinated limb movements, and even cognitive functions involving time judgments.

The basal ganglia are a set of subcortical nuclei deep within the brain. If the cerebellum is important for the timing of movements and thoughts, the basal ganglia are essential for starting, stopping, and shifting between them.

Like the cerebellum, they connect the cortex to the brainstem and spinal cord via the relay centers of the thalamus. Input to the basal ganglia comes from multiple areas of the cerebral cortex, including the motor, limbic, and prefrontal areas. This input follows a circumscribed circuit within the basal ganglia from the input nuclei (the *caudate* and *putamen*, together known as the *striatum*) to the output nuclei and then back to the cortical area from which it started, as well as to the spinal cord.

There are two key concepts regarding the basal ganglia. First, as you may have guessed, the individual nuclei are somatotopically organized throughout the entire circuit. For example, input from the left arm region of the right supplementary motor cortex will stay segregated through the striatum and arrive back to the left arm region of the right supplementary motor cortex via the thalamus.

Second, like the cerebellum, the basal ganglia use two channels of opposite polarity: the 'direct' activating and 'indirect' inhibitory pathways from the substantia nigra to the putamen. Both pathways are mediated by dopamine, but have opposite effects because they work through two different dopamine receptors. The direct pathway involves the D1 dopamine receptor, while the indirect pathway uses the D2 receptor. These opposing signals embrace each other in a neural ballet, producing an intricate downstream cascade and turning on and off other neurons as they twirl through the various parts of the basal ganglia, the thalamus, and on to the motor cortex. The dopamine dance is necessary to maintain the proper balance between movement and stasis, approach and withdrawal, impulse and apathy. We hardly take notice of this subcortical celebration when all is going well, but sometimes the music stops.

Parkinson's disease is caused by the destruction of dopaminergic neurons in the substantia nigra through drugs, toxins, repeated head trauma, or some unknown mechanism. This results in the preferential activation of the indirect pathway in the nigrostriatal dopamine system, which in turn leads to the inhibition of voluntary movements. Parkinson patients experience progressive difficulty in movement initiation and a poverty of movement amplitude and speed. In the early stages, cognition remains intact. But as the disease progresses, the ability to shift from thought to thought, an essential component of human mental life, is adversely affected.

One way to look at the situation in the basal ganglia is that dopamine functions as a motivational signal that primes ongoing motor circuits to anticipate the next step. Just as dopamine tags reward onto novel stimuli in the cognitive sphere, so too does it function in the realm of motion, where the concept of *reward* is defined as the successful execution of the requisite movement.

From Motion to Cognition

The basal ganglia connect to various regions of the cortex through the mesocortical and mesolimbic dopamine systems. These include areas responsible for emotion (*medial* and *orbitofrontal regions*), planning (the *dorsilateral prefrontal regions*), and judgment (the *anterior cingulate cortex*). Cortical input from a specific site is processed by the corresponding part of the basal ganglia and returned, via the thalamus, to the place from which it came, in neatly segregated 'cortico-striato-thalamo-cortical' loops. Diseases of mood and cognition such as bipolar disorder, obsessive-compulsive disorder, attention deficit disorder, schizophrenia, and autism may all involve pathology in some region of the basal ganglia. Perhaps these defects are linked to neurochemical imbalances in nonmotor cortico-striatal circuits, just as Parkinson's disease results from imbalances in the motor circuits. Balanced activity between the direct and indirect pathways may be necessary for *conscious shifting* between actions, moods, and decisions. If so, an overactive direct pathway in the basal ganglia will result in hyperactive motion, emotion, or cognition, while an overactive indirect pathway results in lethargy, depression, and psychomotor retardation.

The basal ganglia and cerebellum form two distinct modulatory loops within the larger sensory-motor loop. The basal ganglia allow the individual to shift between acts, moods, and thoughts. The cerebellum is a fine-tuning machine that filters sensory-motor activity to produce smoother, better synchronized motions and thoughts. These two structures, working through the thalamus, help integrate the perceptual stream with the motor stream.

Practice Makes Perfect

Much of what we do each day is routine. We wake up, get out of bed, and drag a comb across our head without much thought. These actions don't require much in the way of executive control; indeed, it would be a waste of mental resources if we had to exercise attention and willpower each time we comb our hair. There is also much experimental evidence that paying attention to actions that are normally performed well without conscious thought causes *deterioration* in performance. Professional athletes and actors are all too familiar with this phenomenon, popularly known as 'choking'.

Just as memories are slowly transferred from the hippocampus to the cortex, learned actions are gradually transferred from the cortex to the basal ganglia as they become habitual. Recall that the basal ganglia form parallel circuit loops with the cortex. Specific motor or cognitive functions such as the ability to whistle a tune or perform simple arithmetic are mapped onto a corresponding area of the basal ganglia. Motor routines appear to be preferentially mapped to a part of the basal ganglia called the putamen, while cognitive routines are mapped to the caudate nucleus.

The basal ganglia are important in the establishment of learned routines and habits. They relieve the cortex from having to attend to mundane activity. Additionally, they integrate the components of habits into a smooth operation. The neuroscientist Ann Graybiel has proposed that the basal ganglia re-codes cortical inputs into chunks of sequential behavior. Thus, once we have learned to swim, we don't have to think, 'left arm stroke, right arm stroke, head turn, BREATHE!…' We simply go with the flow and swim without having to think about it at all. Once a cortical-basal ganglia loop is selected, the entire ensemble is expressed as a chunk. Normally, we have control over the deployment of these automatic loops. We can decide when to swim or stop swimming, how fast, in which direction, and so on. These are top-down signals from the frontal cortex. But there are two well known disorders in which conscious control of habitual behavior is derailed: *Gilles de la Tourette's syndrome* (*TS*) and *obsessive compulsive disorder* (*OCD*).

TS is characterized by repeated 'tics': abrupt movements or vocalizations that resemble fragments of purposeful behavior. People with TS may suddenly jerk their arms, clear their throats, or even utter obscenities. These are not fully willed actions; the individual is helpless to suppress the urge to tic, which is often exacerbated by stress and fatigue. Although such urges can be voluntarily suppressed for periods of time, they must ultimately be released as 'a swimmer needs to come up for air', as one TS sufferer put it.

OCD and its cousins, obsessive-compulsive personality trait, hypochondrias, and the various body dysmorphic disorders such as anorexia nervosa and bulimia, are characterized by unwanted thoughts or obsessions such as the nagging feeling that one's body or environment is unclean, unhealthy, or somehow not right. To ameliorate these obsessions, the sufferer compulsively repeats ritualistic behaviors to reduce the anxiety (washing one's hands, checking the locks, hoarding old newspapers, demanding blood tests, bingeing and purging) dozens or hundreds of times.

TS and OCD share some similarities. As many as 90% of TS individuals also have some characteristics of OCD. Both disorders involve urges to engage in repetitive, ritualistic and otherwise unwanted behavior. In both cases, the behavior can be consciously suppressed for some time. The neural link between the disorders is the cortical-basal ganglia loop mentioned earlier. TS is caused by up-regulation of the *motor loop* that connects the putamen with motor and verbal regions of the parietal lobe, while OCD is believed to be due to over-activation of the *cognitive loop* that links the caudate with cognitive regions of the frontal lobe. Chunks of habits and thoughts come rushing to the surface, overwhelming the normal censorship imposed by the cortex. Individuals with TS and OCD effectively become stuck doing things and thinking thoughts that are no longer appropriate or adaptive to the contingencies at hand. In these disorders much conscious control is lost, leading to repetition and perseveration.

OCD is commonly treated with a combination of anti-anxiety medications, which interfere with the hyperactive dopamine neurons, and cognitive psychotherapy, which trains the conscious mind to better suppress unwanted compulsions. But for some patients, this is not enough. Brain surgery is another option for those with severe refractory disease. The thinking here is that if the circuits linking the subcortical source of the unwanted dopamine is physically severed from rational parts of the brain which fabricates the obsessions, then the behavior will go away. Psychosurgery has had a mixed track record. The frontal lobotomies performed so casually in the middle of the last century for all sorts of psychiatric disorders often 'cured' disabling symptoms of psychosis, depression, and compulsions. But by removing dopamine's all-important motivational signal, these procedures frequently left their recipients severely lethargic and apathetic. Newer techniques are now being employed that are more precise and selective in targeting specific unwanted circuits while leaving most other connections alone. These involve microsurgery to the *internal capsule* connecting the basal ganglia with the frontal cortex, implantation of electrodes that reversibly impede subcortical signals, and targeted beams of radiation (*gamma knife)* that converge on specific parts of the cortico-striatal circuit.

Flow and Inspiration

Individuals with TS and OCD often report that the worst part of their conditions is having to deal with social stigma and the circumscribed demands of everyday life. The disappointment of knowing that they spend so much of their time and energy on inappropriate and wasteful rituals leads to mental anguish. But left to their own devices, they could happily engage in their ritualistic tics and compulsions all day, every day. So why do pointless tics and compulsions feel so good for them? Consider this question: why do so many of us enjoy recreational dancing, singing, walking, and swimming? To an anthropologist from Mars, they are equally pointless and repetitive. The answer lies in dopamine.

Whenever we lose ourselves in rhythm, from dancing to throat clearing to hair twirling, dopamine is released in the basal ganglia. This doesn't cause happiness; *it is happiness.* Mihaly Csikszentmihalyi, the author of <u>Flow</u>, believes that some of our happiest moments come from rehearsing well-learned tasks over and over. The repeated stimulation of dopaminergic neurons triggers the reward centers of our brains. It doesn't really matter what sets them off as long as they're activated. In that sense, the only difference between leisure activities like dancing and pathological behavior like tics is the court of social convention.

Another curious aspect of semi-automatic repetitive behavior is its association with inspiration. How many times have you sat down to your computer or trudged off to the library a few days before a big term paper deadline determined to get some last minute inspiration? If you're like most people, you've probably sat down for hours, getting distracted by anything on the web and everyone in the immediate vicinity, coming up with great ideas for everything from your next vacation to finding a perfect Christmas gift, and finally left with nothing but an empty notebook, frustration, and despair. But you can probably also recall many instances where great ideas just popped into your head out of the blue when you were least expecting it. Strangely, these moments often occur in the middle of automatic routines, like taking a shower or tending the garden.

I believe that inspiration often starts subconsciously, fermenting for some time beneath the cortex, making connections with activated regions near and far, before bubbling up to the surface to surprise the interpreter in the left hemisphere. So it may feel to you (the interpreter) as if the creative idea just popped out of nowhere, but really it was there all along, just waiting for the opportune time to come up. The left hemisphere is normally so busy figuring out what to attend to and concocting a coherent story out of the constant sensory stream rushing in, that it can't afford to focus in on whatever bits of ideas may be floating around in the right hemisphere or in the basal ganglia. Investing in imaginary ideas that may never pan out is too risky, so the cortex simply keeps them suppressed.

The left hemisphere can be seduced, however, by repetitive activity generated by the mesocortical dopamine system. When the interpreter is distracted by reward signals from below, it lets go of its hold on the basal ganglia and the right hemisphere. This allows the ideas stored in those regions to enter consciousness as inspiration and creativity. If you really want to do a good job on that term paper, group project, or grant proposal, consider going for a long brisk walk or a dance club first. You might be pleasantly surprised.

Hothead

Pleasure, pain, ecstasy, anxiety, despondency, anger, fear, apprehension, remorse, jealousy, *schadenfreude*, the seven deadly sins: all are part of the human emotional repertoire. We encounter people and situations every day that make us feel and express any of a variety of emotions. But what is emotion, exactly? There are *emotions*, and then there are *feelings*. These terms are so familiar to us that we use them interchangeably in casual speech. But for our more formal purposes they refer to two quite different things. Emotions are visceral signals that refer to the physical state of arousal produced by a particular stimulus. They are the body states caused by the action of the autonomic nervous system and parts of the endocrine system, which together oversee the regulatory activities necessary for life. The rapid heartbeat and breathing, clammy hands, and dry mouth some of us experience before taking an exam constitute *anxiety*, a familiar emotion. But it is the conscious elaboration of this emotion makes it a 'feeling'. Feelings are cortical expressions of underlying subconscious emotional states. Both are necessary for guiding our behavior.

Contrary to common belief and intuition, feelings usually come from emotions, rather than the other way around. The great American psychologist William James got it exactly right over a century ago when he wrote, 'we feel sorry because we cry, angry because we strike, afraid because we tremble and not that we cry, strike or tremble because we are sorry, angry or fearful as the case may be.' Of course, thinking sad thoughts can make us cry, and dwelling on past injustices can make us angry, but more often it is the subconscious emotional state that brings feelings to the surface.

Emotions evolved in our animal ancestors because they are useful for survival. Organisms use them to represent and communicate information about the most basic drives of life: food, sex, and health. Humans can elaborate emotions into feeling states, which allow better perception and control of social behavior. Emotions are the domain of a part of the brain called the *limbic system*, which evolved with the first mammals over 200 million years ago. All mammals have limbic structures in their brains, presumably to facilitate the communication demands of a warm-blooded, fast-paced lifestyle. Emotional expression allows social animals to reveal their needs and desires to themselves and to others in compact, abstract form. In effect, emotions function as pattern detectors. Rats, cats, and bats all display anger, fear, and surprise through facial expressions designed to be readily visible to others of their species. Organisms that are capable of these expressions can convey much more information about their physical and biological state than those that are not. Reptiles and fish rely on more direct, less symbolic signals to achieve these ends. They eat and they sleep, and often see and hear exceptionally well. But fish and reptile eyes are cold. Unlike mammals, they are devoid of emotion. Let's examine the anatomy and physiology of the limbic system before moving on to the construction of human feelings.

The key component in emotional processing is the *amygdala*, a small ovoid structure deep within the medial temporal lobe on each side of the brain. The amygdala receives raw sensory input (visual, auditory, somatosensory) in one of two ways, either directly through the brain's great relay station, the thalamus, or preprocessed via the cerebral cortex. If the input is emotionally significant, such as the sight of a snake, which seems to trigger an innate fear circuit in baby brains, or the roar of a fire engine, the amygdala is aroused and sends an activating signal to the *hypothalamus*. The hypothalamus, in turn, activates the *sympathetic system*, part of the *autonomic* or 'automatic' nervous system, which increases heart rate and blood pressure, and dilates the pupils, preparing the individual for action. This is the so-called fight or flight response. At higher levels of negative emotional arousal, the *parasympathetic system* (another part of the autonomic nervous system) is also activated, producing contractions of smooth muscles leading to the rather unpleasant loss of bowel and bladder control. With sustained anxiety, the hypothalamus instructs the endocrine system to secrete corticosteroids (the stress hormones), which have multiple, far ranging actions on the body, including down-regulation of the immune system and changes in salt and potassium balance. In effect, the long-term health of the body is sacrificed for enhanced short-term performance.

The amygdala is necessary for attaching emotional tags or *valences* onto particular stimuli or situations that may be appetitive or aversive. Some of these associations, such as the fear of snakes, are genetically preprogrammed. But most must be learned through conditioning. Experiments have demonstrated that rats learn to associate the pairing of a neutral stimulus, such as a tone, with a negative one, an electric shock, quite easily. This learning is abolished when the animals have their amygdala removed. Once the initial learning or conditioning phase is completed, and the emotion is bound to the corresponding perception of the object or situation, the emotional trace or memory is stored in the amygdala or the surrounding cerebral cortex. Whenever the creature subsequently finds itself in a similar situation, it automatically and unconsciously generates the appropriate emotional response. In humans, many of the emotions generated by the amygdala are transferred up to the cortex where they enter the realm of awareness and become feelings to be utilized for social judgment and behavior.

The dual channel pathway is adaptive in that the fast subcortical/ subconscious pathway can prime the amygdala to receive more refined cortical/ conscious input a split-second later. This may form the basis for the *priming effect* seen in many psychological experiments where a stimulus that is flashed too rapidly for conscious registration nonetheless affects conscious judgment. In addition, the amygdala's role in memory consolidation is distinct from that played by the hippocampus. The hippocampus is the gateway for episodic memories (what you had for breakfast this morning) and semantic knowledge (London is the capital of England) to enter their respective repositories in the temporal lobes. On the other hand, the consolidation of emotional memories (the experience of being mugged on the subway) requires the amygdala. The two memory systems appear to be dissociable. The famous patient, H.M., who suffered profound amnesia after having both of his hippocampi surgically removed in a botched attempt to correct his epilepsy, could not recall the scientists who greeted him every morning. Yet he had a vague feeling that one of them was more pleasant than the other. This was because H.M. could still record emotional memories through his intact amygdala.

The major input channels to the amygdala, both directly from the thalamus, or indirectly via the cortex, are multimodal sensory (sight, sound, touch, taste, smell). The output from the amygdala is also twofold. First there is the descending channel to the hypothalamus and brainstem responsible for the emotional response (fight or flight). Second, there is an ascending channel to the limbic cortex, which produces feelings. The limbic cortex refers to several regions in the front or *prefrontal* part of the brain, which receive massive connections from the amygdala. The prefrontal cortex is the largest and most highly evolved part of the primate brain. It is responsible for the calculations and decisions that facilitate rational thought and social judgment, namely those attributes we commonly refer to as 'intelligence'.

In summary, the amygdala plays three roles. First, it is the organ of *emotional perception*, receiving salient input from both the thalamus and the cortex. Second, it is the engine of *emotional learning and memory*, conferring emotional valence on conditioned stimuli and storing it in the cortex. Finally, it is the source of *emotional expression*, generating the autonomic, behavioral, and endocrine changes associated with anxiety. The output from the amygdala via the hypothalamus and the autonomic nervous system bathes every tissue of the body, preparing it for whatever action contingency it may encounter. But the activation signal is nonspecific. The pulse quickens equally whether one beholds a hungry lion, a parking ticket, or a beautiful blind date. Humans do not simply show emotion, but also ask why they are feeling it. For this to happen, the expressed emotion itself needs to be perceived and interpreted by the cortex.

Signals from the emotionally aroused body are coded by sensory fibers throughout the gut and the circulatory and respiratory systems and directed up the spinal cord, through the brainstem, and on into the thalamus. There, a crude somatotopic map is constructed representing the activation pattern of the body. This information is then shunted to a primitive cortical region hidden deep within the interior surface of the Sylvian fissure on either side. These are the *insulae*. Each insula (left and right) has its own somatotopic map representing the opposite side of the body. Emotional information is elaborated here after its projection from the thalamus. Neurons of the insula are exquisitely sensitive to negative emotions like pain, hunger, and fear. The insula, especially on the right side, starts the process of emotional interpretation that reaches its climax in the prefrontal cortex and the anterior cingulate.

The insula is an evolutionarily ancient structure, but it and the nearby anterior cingulate cortex to which it projects are endowed with a surfeit of a relatively new (in evolutionary terms) type of nerve cell, the *von Economo spindle neuron* (*VEN*). These cells have unusually large dendritic territories and long axons that collect and transmit information through wide swaths of the brain. Furthermore, they are found only in the great apes, and are ten-fold more common in humans than in chimpanzees and gorillas. It is possible that the VENs are the neural substrate that permit the uniquely human ability to link body-state perceptions with affective cognition.

Recently, neuroscientists have used fMRI scanners to image the brains of people experiencing *envy* and *schadenfreude*. When participants were instructed to imagine someone blessed with undeserved good fortune, increased metabolic activity was found in the fusiform gyrus, the amygdala, the insula, the prefrontal and anterior cingulate areas, and the somatosensory regions responsible for pain perception. This fits in quite nicely with the affective circuits I proposed earlier.

The neural correlate of envy may go something like this. First, seeing (or imagining, as the case my be) the subject of your envy activates your temporal lobe's fusiform face discrimination zone. If this face has been associated with emotional saliency from prior experience, your amygdala is activated. Efferent signals are then sent down to the hypothalamus, which turns on the sympathetic nervous system, making you sweat, raising your pulse and blood pressure, clenching your jaw muscles, and so on. Your fight or flight response (the emotion) is then picked up by the thalamus, projected to the insula, and then on to the orbitofrontal and anterior cingulate regions of the frontal lobe. This visceral input is also sent up to the cortical regions that represent pain. There is also a more direct route from the amygdala straight to the frontal regions, bypassing the hypothalamus/body loop. The orbitofrontal and anterior cingulate regions of the cerebral cortex take the emotional raw material coming in from the insula and use it to weave a conscious narrative of the feeling of envy.

One curious aspect concerns the activation of pain processing centers of the cortex. Envy doesn't exactly cause the somatic kind of physical pain one would experience from a gunshot wound. But the visceral receptors are activated just the same and relay this information to body maps in the somatosensory cortex. It seems that the frontal cortex uses this representation of pain in the sensory cortex to re-create a sense of 'what it must be like' to actually be in pain.

The felt experience is simply the final, or rather, the latest, draft written by the interpreter. As new information arrives through the amygdala and the insula loops, the cortex constantly updates its activation patterns. Through each revision, the narrative acquires more nuance, definition, and meaning. The undifferentiated emotional state represented by the autonomic nervous system gradually becomes something more focused, specific, and compelling; first a vague perception of unease, then a definite sense of indignation, and eventually a full blown feeling of 'I hate this guy, he's not better than me, he's not smarter than me, why should he deserve his million dollar salary, his fast cars, and his beautiful girlfriends??!!'

Imaging studies on envy's sister *schadenfreude* (the wonderful German word referring to the taking of pleasure in others' misfortunes) have revealed similar activation patterns with one difference: instead of the pain regions of the somatosensory cortex, the reward circuits of the basal ganglia seem to light up. This likely correlates with activation of the mesocortial and mesolimbic dopamine systems, producing feelings of satisfaction. I predict that the other six deadly sins: lust, gluttony, greed, sloth, pride, and wrath would activate similar brain areas. The first five are 'appetitive' sins, like *schadenfreude*, and are likely to activate the dopamine circuits. The last one, wrath, is more akin to the negative feeling of envy, and involves activity in the pain areas.

Love and Oxytocin

Dopamine is not the only neurotransmitter that affects emotion and decision-making. The hypothalamus synthesizes a pair of nine residue polypeptide hormones called *oxytocin* and *vasopressin*. Vasopressin, also known as *anti-diuretic hormone*, is released in response to decreased osmotic concentration in the blood. It acts to constrict blood vessels and increase the resorption of water in the kidney, resulting in higher blood pressure. This was an adaptive mechanism for our ancestors who often suffered from dehydration or traumatic blood loss. The related hormone oxytocin is released by females during and immediately after childbirth, causing uterine contractions and the 'letdown reflex' of breast milk into the lactiferous ducts. These two hormones and their receptors are believed to have diverged from a common pair of ancestral genes that first evolved in primitive fish about 500 million years ago.

More relevant for our discussion is oxytocin's role in cognitive psychology. It is known that the hormone is found in greater concentrations in the blood of both sexes just after orgasms associated with sexual intercourse. Animals studies have found that it fosters pair bonding and monogamy. And there is now recent evidence that it mediates trust and empathy, as well. What appears to be happening is that oxytocin dampens the amygdala's natural tendency to generate anxiety. This is important for reproductive success; imagine how disastrous it would be for the species if females rejected a potential mate's every advance. A squirt of oxytocin into the limbic system inhibits the hypothalamic-pituitary stress response, and facilitates affection between mother and child, and husband and wife.

Interestingly, inborn variations in the *oxytocin receptor* (OXTR) gene appear to underlie certain personality traits. In a recent study, psychologist Sarina Rodrigues and her colleagues have identified two common OXTR variants. People with two copies of the *A* variant tended to do worse on tests of empathy and social understanding, better on tests of analytical reasoning, described themselves as more anxious and less affectionate, and were more likely to be autistic than those with two copies of the *G* variant.

How can one neurotransmitter generate such diversity of response? The answer lies in receptor specificity and downstream modulation. Different tissues express different concentrations of the oxytocin receptor. The nipple, the uterus, and the *nucleus accumbens* of the brain have more of them per volume than the spleen or the pancreas. And the cells in these tissues also express a wide range of different transcription factors that work to turn on or off many genes in various combinations in response to the same oxytocin signal from above. There is nothing particularly special about the size and shape of the oxytocin molecule; what's important is how it's used. It is a reflection of the economy of natural selection that one random polypeptide happened to be chosen for so many vital roles in physiology, psychology, and behavior.

Egghead

Over the last ten million years of primate evolution, one part of the brain has ballooned in size more than any other, reaching near comical proportions in the human animal. It is the prefrontal cortex (PFC), a collection of brain tissue encompassing three functional subdivisions: the *dorsolateral* (DLPFC), *ventromedial* (VMPFC), and *orbitofrontal* (OFC) areas. In humans, the PFC takes up nearly a third of the cortex, requiring an enormous skull case that often endangers the lives of mother and offspring alike during childbirth. Even so, all babies are born with brains still woefully premature. Just as the PFC was the latest part of the human brain to develop in evolutionary terms, so too is it the last part to mature in developmental terms. Its neurons are not fully insulated until late adolescence. This is the main reason why teenagers otherwise physically and sexually mature exhibit such poor judgment, attention, and self-control. They may be intelligent beyond their years and wickedly proficient at text messaging, but their behavior is more often akin to that of wild animals trapped in their narrow here and now. Policy makers and parents would be wise to keep this in mind when entrusting young people with adult responsibilities like alcohol, motor vehicles, and credit cards.

The PFC stands at the apex of cognition, judgment, and decision-making. It may not be central to phenomenal consciousness, but it plays the leading role in what we commonly define as 'intelligence'. So let's explore how this marvelous organ works, starting with the lateral component. The DLPFC receives a massive amount of input from all over the brain, especially the sensory association areas that hold high-level representations of visual, auditory, and somatosensory perceptions. It sends output fibers into the high-order motor areas that contain representations of complex motor commands. In addition, the DLPFC has reciprocal connections with many subcortical regions including the thalamus, hippocampus, basal ganglia, and cerebellum. These connections allow neural networks in the lateral PFC to represent schemas and action plans that encompass multiple modalities (locomotion, gaze, language). Unlike activation patterns in the distal end of the motor pathway, prefrontal schemas are highly abstract.

The purpose of the DLPFC is twofold. First, it is important for motor learning, especially for behaviors that contain multiple sub-components, each of which requires the focusing and shifting of attention. Changing a flat tire for the first time would be a good example. Second, it is necessary for actions that require the maintenance of attention, especially in the face of interruption and delay. Lab monkeys whose PFC's were deactivated (by cooling) demonstrated failure to adequately shift and maintain attention for goal-directed behaviors. The common feature here is control of cortical ensembles over time. In other parts of the brain, such as the primary motor strip, the visual cortex, or the thalamus, activation patterns are relatively transient and prone to capture by bottom-up influences from the dynamically changing neural environment around them. But PFC activation patterns are more durable. This allows it to encode neural patterns corresponding to complex learned behaviors. In fact, the DLPFC exerts a major top-down modulatory influence on motor control.

The control of timing in motor function is as important as the representation of space in sensory perception. So much of our behavior requires that we deploy our actions in precisely the right sequence at the right time, and we usually don't know how things are going until the action is well underway. But with practice, we can *anticipate* the contingencies to the point that it becomes almost automatic. This happens once we learn how to uncork a wine bottle, swing a tennis racquet, or write a cheque. Overlearned behaviors shift activation from conscious control in the PFC to subcortical areas like the basal ganglia and the cerebellum.

The ability to hold plans in short-term working memory (for up to a minute in monkeys) while engaging in an unrelated activity is part of what psychologists call *executive function* (EF). EF's also include the ability to multitask, resist distracters, and shift attention depending on changing contingencies. The basis of EF is a top-down signal from the PFC to the effecter regions that inhibit prepotent responses.

The first step involves priming the PFC with reward signals through the mesocortical dopamine pathway. Stimuli that possess these motivational tags prompt the assembly of dynamic PFC networks representing goals. These networks then project to the motor areas where they strengthen current representations, protect them from degradation, and provide activating signals that bias processing towards the task at hand.

In contrast to the DLPFC, the nearby VMPFC and OFC are intimately connected to the limbic structures, and are therefore more involved in emotional processing. But their functional architecture is quite similar. They support neural networks that code not for any particular aspect of an object or event, but rather for the cues and contingencies associated with salient stimuli. And like the lateral PFC, these zones modulate the activity of motor regions through top-down signals. These three regions work together in the human brain, allowing it to create associations used not just for coordinating motions, but also for feeling emotions with a richness that no other animal can match. And, as we shall see in the next section, emotional perceptions are crucial for complex cognition and judgment.

The cardinal virtues of patience, perseverance, focus, flexibility, insight, clarity, creativity, quickness of thought, and wit are all products of a healthy PFC. Their power and magic are perhaps best seen in the mind of our remarkable and promising young president, Barack Obama. It would be instructive to image President Obama's brain. I'm willing to bet that his limbic-prefrontal circuits light up vigorously when making crucial decisions like getting bipartisan support for Wall Street financial reform and international cooperation on corralling loose enriched uranium stockpiles. Obama's preternaturally calm and collected demeanor, his uncanny ability to deliberately step outside of his immediate environment and reflect on the big picture from a distance, his fluency in thinking about his own thinking, something psychologists have called *metacognition*, and, not least, his fluidity on the basketball court are likely to show up as activation in his subcortical brain areas such as the basal ganglia and cerebellum. And as a left-hander, he may even recruit unusual support from the gestalt-laden right hemisphere.

But just as important in Obama's executive control is one last secret weapon in his neural armamentarium: a mechanism that harnesses the raw power of his entire body's emotional state to the full computational capacity of his lateral prefrontal cortex.

Just Do It

Perhaps the most celebrated case in the annals of neuroscience was that of Phineas Gage, a railroad construction worker who in 1848 was freakishly injured by an explosion on the job. The blast hurled a metal rod into his face, which impaled his left cheekbone, bored through his brain, and exited through the top of his skull landing several dozen feet away. Remarkably, Gage soon regained consciousness and actually 'recovered' within a few months. This is where the story really gets interesting.

By most contemporary accounts, Gage was a sober and responsible individual before his mishap. But afterwards, people noticed that his personality and behavior had changed. He became increasingly irritable, irresponsible with his finances, and impulsive in his vocational choices. Gage joined the Barnum and Bailey circus, traveled the country with his famous metal rod at his side, lost his earnings to gambling and unscrupulous business associates, and generally led a rootless existence until his death 13 years later from seizures related to his head injury.

In 1994, neuroanatomist Hanna Damasio used Gage's skull (housed at the Harvard Medical School Museum) and state-of-the-art neuroimaging software to recreate the brain lesion in question. The metal rod was found to have neatly excavated a cylindrical volume of brain tissue encompassing most of Gage's OFC, VMPFC, and some parts of his DLPFC on both sides, miraculously sparing all the regions responsible for memory, speech, movement, and sensation.

In his landmark book, <u>Descartes' Error</u>, neurologist Antonio Damasio describes one of his own patients whom he calls a 'modern day Phineas Gage'. Elliot was diagnosed with a brain tumor that originated between the two frontal lobes and gradually compressed his VMPFC's bilaterally. Like Gage, Elliot suffered no sensory, motor, or perceptual impairment. In addition, his working memory appeared intact (he scored above average on standard tests of executive function). But unlike Gage, Elliot was not prone to impulsivity and emotional outbursts. On the contrary, he became extremely *indecisive*. Instructed to go to the grocery and pick up some breakfast items, Elliot would take forever endlessly mulling over the pros and cons of each and every brand of cereal and orange juice. Unable to make efficient decisions, Elliot eventually lost his job and his savings.

The curious cases of Gage and Elliot demonstrate the intimate relationship between reason and emotion in the decision-making sphere. Antonio Damasio has articulated a model that gives a parsimonious explanation for this relationship that is grounded in neuroanatomy and physiology: *the somatic marker hypothesis.*

Let's review: the 'images' generated by sensory perception and, to a lesser extent, those generated internally as imagination arrive in the amygdala, which then passes them along to the rest of the body via the hypothalamus and the autonomic nervous system. The resulting *emotional state* can then be perceived and interpreted by the cortex via the insula as *feelings.* Damasio calls this circuit the 'body-loop'. Recall that there is a second, more direct route from amygdala to cortex that also produces conscious feelings of a sort without having to go through the rest of the body. Damasio call this the 'as-if body loop', but I like to call it the 'brain loop.' Feelings in the brain do not require the body to experience the emotions to make them real. A stimulus laden with emotional valence can be processed directly by the cortex without a first pass through the body. But those feelings generated by the brain loop are qualitatively inferior to those produced by the body loop. Emotions heighten whatever it is one is thinking. On the other hand, emotions will become stronger without thoughts to inhibit them. It is the body loop that produces the somatic markers: the emotions associated with difficult choices that help us decide between them. The body and brain loops converge in the VMPFC to produce the feelings necessary to expedite the decision-making process.

Damasio describes somatic markers as a dynamic portrait of the organism's physiological state that is represented and re-represented in successively higher processing areas: thalamus, insula, somatosensory cortex, and VMPFC. In the end, the rational decision maker in the lateral PFC gets to 'view' and evaluate these pictures coming from the body, compare them with the action schemas they activate via the dopamine system, and come up with a recommendation for the motor areas.

I would like to expand the somatic marker hypothesis to the amygdala. The dopamine value system in the amydala that signals anticipation and reward activates the PFC. But the PFC feeds back to the amygdala and inhibits it, a well known process called *frontal inhibition.* In fact, cortical activity in general suppresses the amygdala. This is because the major neurotransmitter receptor in the amygdala, the *GABA receptor*, hyperpolarizes (turns off) its neuron. When axons from the cortex or brainstem fire onto dendrites in the amygdala, they activate the GABA receptors, which then decrease the usual amount of activity there. On the other hand, when there is a lack of incoming activity, the amygdala tends to become more excited. The amygdala turns up the cortex, but the cortex turns down the amygdala, or to put it more bluntly, *emotions promote thought, but thoughts keep the emotions in check.* If the PFC is dysfunctional or immature, feedback inhibition to the amygdala is lost in a phenomenon known as *frontal release.* This is why babies and young children, individuals with ADHD or autism, and the elderly who suffer from Alzheimers disease are so emotionally labile.

Armed with this knowledge of neuroscience, we can begin to differentiate the psychological characteristics exhibited by Phineas Gage and Elliot. I propose that Gage's deficits can be explained by his larger area of brain damage. His traumatic brain injury disrupted all limbic modulation. As a result, his amygdala was disinhibited and juiced up his body and the rest of his cortex. The ability to plan for the future and suppress primal emotions was lost, explaining his anxiety and impulsiveness. His actions were driven not by long-term plans for minimizing pain or maximizing pleasure, but rather by the immediate gratification of the goal at hand. Additionally, Gage probably also suffered deficits in organization, concentration, and memory retrieval due to additional damage to the working memory centers in the DLPFC.

Elliot's psychological profile was quite different from Gage's. First, he became more indecisive rather than impulsive, yet he still made poor judgments. Second, his affect became markedly blunted. Third, he was generally less anxious and hotheaded. Fourth, he had no significant difficulty with working memory. These findings can be explained by neuroanatomy. Elliot's lesion was more circumscribed to the OFC and the VMPFC, sparing the working memory centers of the DLPFC. Thus frontal inhibition of the amygdala could still take place, preventing limbic overload (impulsivity, anxiety, violent temper tantrums). However, emotional valence could not be coupled to the decision-making process. His somatic markers were no longer there for him to make gut decisions. Elliot became indecisive and hyper-rational. He tended to overanalyze all possible consequences of potential actions prior to making his (usually poor) decisions. According to the somatic marker hypothesis, we have evolved to allow our subconscious neural patterns to access the conscious parts of our brains and bias our decision making process. This is useful in making life and death choices in the heat of the moment – choices that our limited working memory would never be able to make on its own.

In effect, Phineas Gage's decision-making was driven by system one, while Elliott's was driven by system two. Good decisions require both systems working in tandem. As revealed in the priming and embodied cognition experiments I described earlier, we humans chronically overestimate the capacity of system two and underestimate the power of system one. My own system one led me to risk my life by plunging thousands of feet into a meadow at Interlaken.

Chapter 3

Religion

NO GOD, NO PEACE
KNOW GOD, KNOW PEACE

Right wing bumper sticker

KNOW GOD, NO PEACE
NO GOD, KNOW PEACE

Left wing bumper sticker

Religion is a desperate measure that people resort to when the stakes are high and they have exhausted the usual techniques for the causation of success-medicines, strategies, courtship, and, in the case of the weather, nothing.

Steven Pinker
How the Mind Works

I wanted all things
To seem to make some sense
So that we could all be happy, yes,
Instead of tense.
And I make up lies
So they all fit nice,
And I make this sad world
A Par-a-dise.

Kurt Vonnegut, Jr
Cat's Cradle

Religion is uniquely human and so widespread across cultures, like language, like consciousness, that it positively begs an explanation. I'm not interested in debating the existence of God or the probability of an afterlife, nor am I interested in discussing the authenticity of holy texts. As a scientifically minded atheist, I will assume that these are all the products of human imagination. What holds my interest is the very root of religion: the belief in magical thought. In this chapter, I will put forth a novel theory on the origins of religion that incorporates evolutionary, neuroscientific, and cultural perspectives.

All religions and the cults from which they started are cultural phenomena whose particular doctrines and rituals have been fabricated by people, not by God. But the tendency of people to become religious probably has a genetic basis. How else to explain its universality? Like love and lust, language and color vision, the capacity for religion may be innately programmed into our minds by the genes that build our brains.

Religion provokes controversy. I'm not talking about the struggle between fundamentalists of various stripes who seek to infect society with their own brand of militant theocracy and liberals who defend secular democracy with equal passion. There is another less-publicized debate going on up in the ivory towers of academia. It concerns the evolutionary foundations of religion as a 'natural phenomenon'. On one side of the divide are scholars who believe religion evolved for a reason: it helped ancestors who were endowed with brains capable of magical thought to survive and produce more like-minded offspring. They maintain that magical thinking itself is heritable and confers a selective advantage. On the other side are those who believe that religion is not particularly adaptive. Moreover, they maintain that religion is not in our genes; it is a cultural phenomenon that is a by-product of the complexity of our minds. But such by-products themselves can evolve in much the same way that genes do, competing for space in our minds like some insidious parasite. I will examine the merits of both positions in this nature/nurture debate on the origins of religion. But first we will need to build up some basic understanding of how the mind works.

From Truth to Knowledge

This is the truth: there is a physical universe out there that our minds cannot directly access. It is a universe made up of particles and force fields governed by the laws of physics and chemistry, and interpretable through the language of mathematics. The universe is big – around 13 billion light years in diameter – and old by human standards, but not infinitely so. We don't know what, if anything, lies outside of its spatial and temporal boundaries (perhaps a plethora of other universes strung out in an infinite nine dimensional 'multiverse' as some string theorists and cosmologists muse?). All we can say for sure is that everything that means anything to us as a species, all the sensations, feelings, memories, pains, joys, desires, and dreams any of us have ever experienced are part of this physical universe and no other. Our bodies, brains, and minds are products of physical laws working through the natural selection of biochemical genes that direct the development of the embryo, the nervous system, and the organization of cognitive modules in the brain.

The scope of physics by definition encompasses the entire universe, but it can only go so far in explaining our subjective experience of the world. This is not because God designed our bodies, or because angels direct our thoughts. Rather, the difficulty stems from our limited subjective perspective. As I discussed in the first chapter, our grasp of the physical world comes necessarily filtered through our senses. We see the world not as it really is, but rather as our brains have been engineered by millions of years of natural selection to perceive it. They are great at creating a useful facsimile or virtual reality model of the outside world. But as all connoisseurs of video games can attest, no matter how good the graphics are, no matter how much they can fool us into believing they are real, once we turn off the monitor and look outside the window, we always realize that they are never as good as the real thing. Something is always lost in the simulation. The trouble is that unlike a video game, we can never turn off the monitor in our brains and cleanse the doors of perception.

The limitations of physics arise because of the sheer complexity that can emerge from the evolution of replicating entities. Biology is a physical process that builds complexity through the evolution of genes. And, as we shall see in the next chapter, culture is a physical process that builds complexity through the evolution of *memes*. At the intersection of biology and culture is psychology, which is itself a physical process that builds complexity through a combination of genes and *memes*. Religion maps onto both psychology and culture, and this is where I shall direct my attention.

How do we know what we know? For thousands of years, this was a question only philosophers dared to tackle, and for thousands of years they stumbled badly, largely because of their addiction to dualism compounded by a stubborn unwillingness to actually dissect the brain. In the last few decades, however, neuroscientists have taken over from the epistemologists by rephrasing the question as: 'how does the brain represent objective reality?' The progress has been dramatic. We now know that semantic knowledge is stored in the neocortex in domain-specific ways; different areas of the cortex are dedicated to particular kinds of concepts, locations, objects, and even faces.

The neuroimaging of people with head injuries has helped scientists map much of the architecture of domain-specific knowledge in the brain. These studies prove that the brain is not an all-purpose black box. Perception flows into recognition and memory in clearly defined neural pathways. For example, when we see an elephant, its various distinguishing properties (long nose, big ears, wrinkly skin, tusks) are encoded in the higher-order visual cortex, whose neurons project to the temporal lobe via the ventral stream. There, neural ensembles that already code for similar features are activated. Within a few hundred milliseconds, a single network representing 'elephant' out-competes other networks representing 'Pinocchio' or 'triceratops' and gets top-bill recruitment into the charmed circle of attention and consciousness. Other networks representing similar compatible concepts such a 'circus' or 'Africa' may also make it into awareness with lesser gusto.

What is remarkable is the organization of *semantic space* in the temporal lobe, the terminus of the ventral stream of visual perception. There is still quite a lot of lively debate among cognitive psychologists as to whether objects are segregated there according to their perceptual properties (colors, shapes, textures, sounds, size, odors) or according to categories (liquid/solid, tool/ weapon, living/inanimate, plant/animal, fruit/vegetable, edible/poisonous). The answer is probably both. Functional MRI studies have identified brain-injured patients who can discriminate among perceptual properties but not categories and vice versa. In the first chapter, we discussed the strange case of prosopagnosia, the inability to recognize familiar faces. In an even more bizarre twist, the British psychologist Elizabeth Warrington conducted a study on a patient who had suffered damage to his temporal lobes (including the fusiform face areas) as a result of several strokes. The patient happened to be a sheep farmer from Herefordshire. He was unable to recognize pictures of famous British politicians, but when shown photos of individual sheep from his own farm, he could identify them perfectly! Other experiments have found patients who were able to discriminate amongst various people and animals, but couldn't tell whether other objects were tools or musical instruments. These studies highlight the ability of the healthy brain to develop very accurate representations of the outside world.

Semantic space is not formless and seamless, like some magic hat from which an infinite number of rabbits can be pulled. It has limits and boundaries that jibe with people, places, and things in the outside world. How else would we make sense of our environment? The blueprint for semantic space is drawn up by brain-building genes that have millions of years of prior experience behind them. Its basic construction is largely completed during embryogenesis and early childhood. The fine-tuning is left for synaptic plasticity. Semantic space does not track reality quite as directly as the retinotopic organization of the visual system or the somatotopic organization of the sensory strip. At first glance, the activity there appears messy, with lots of overlap between perceptual features and subjective categories. But the fact that there is underlying organization is undeniable.

Memories

> Remembering is not the re-excitation of innumerable
> fixed, lifeless and fragmentary traces. It is an imaginative
> reconstruction, or construction, built out of the relation of
> our attitude towards a whole active mass of organized past
> reactions or experience, and to a little outstanding detail
> which commonly appears in image or in language form. It is
> thus hardly ever really exact, even in the most rudimentary
> cases of rote recapitulation, and it is not at all important that
> it should be so.
>
> Sir Frederic Bartlett
> <u>Remembering</u>

Memories come in many varieties: episodic, semantic, procedural, emotional, priming, conditioning, habituation. Episodic and semantic memories are collectively called *explicit memories* because they involve conscious awareness, while the others are referred to as *implicit memories* because they are automatic and subconscious. In the last chapter, we explored emotional memories and priming within the context of system one and the amygdala. Here we will discuss the first three kinds of memory. Episodic or autobiographical memories are the mental reconstructions of specific experiences, such as the taste of your toast this morning or a detail about your date last night. Semantic memories refer to general knowledge of things in the world. It is the knowledge that butter goes well on toast or that you shouldn't ask a woman her age. Procedural memories are the representations the brain uses to carry out a learned behavior, such as spreading butter on toast or kissing your date goodnight.

Both episodic and semantic memories can be subdivided temporally: short (seconds), intermediate (minutes to hours), and long-term (days to years). Short-term memories, such as holding a new phone number in mind long enough to write it down, is actually working memory, which I discussed in the last chapter. It involves transient cortical reverberations at the initial site of processing followed by activation of associated prefrontal areas. The encoding of intermediate and long-term explicit memory, on the other hand, requires a particular subcortical organ in the medial temporal region, the *hippocampus*.

The hippocampi are a pair of seahorse-shaped structures that receive sensory information from the visual, auditory, and somatosensory cortices and store this input within its densely packed neural networks. The neurons of the hippocampus stimulate one another in response to incoming information in a process called *long term potentiation* (LTP), a kind of neural plasticity that involves activity dependent gene expression in the formation of new and durable synaptic junctions. A unique aspect of the hippocampus is that its cells are sensitive to one's position in space. Rodent studies have identified 'place cells' that fire when an animal moves in a specific direction relative to its surroundings and 'grid cells' that fire when it engages a moving object. The neuroscientists Jean Luvet and Josh Sanes have developed an ingenious technique of imaging individual neurons and their axon fibers with brilliant color-coded fluorescent proteins genetically engineered from bioluminescent jellyfish. One such 'brainbow' portrait of mouse hippocampus magnified thousands of times adorns the front cover of this book.

The collective activation patterns of hippocampal cells in response to movement form a code that is useful, and probably essential, for navigation through one's environment. Once encoded, the ensembles corresponding to the contour of a face, the layout of a room, the contents of a suitcase, and whatever other experiences or bits of information one happens to remember are embedded into a preprogrammed coordinate system that roughly represents the viewer's spatial location. These codes are stored for a time in the hippocampus before being gradually transferred into the adjacent cortical areas, where they can become consolidated into long-term memory.

The encoding of experiences into long-term memory involves a journey from the multimodal association cortices, through the medial temporal lobe (semantic space), to the hippocampus proper. From the hippocampus and the other medial temporal areas there are back projections that reenter the cortex. The gradual consolidation of long-term explicit memories into their final resting places in various locations of neocortex depends upon the integrity of the hippocampus, the surrounding cortex, and their input and output projections. The hippocampus is the bridge that links intermediate with long-term storage for both episodic and semantic – but not procedural – memories. Additionally, as we saw in the last chapter, the amygdala plays an important supporting role in the encoding of emotionally salient memories. This is why we tend to remember an emotionally fraught episode so much more clearly than something run-of-the-mill.

Procedural memories do not require the hippocampus for encoding. But they too come in short and long-term flavors. Recent procedural memories are stored directly in the parts of the brain that first mediated the activity. For example, riding a bicycle involves activity in the visual and motor cortex plus the subcortical regions responsible for balance and motor planning: the cerebellum and basal ganglia. With practice, such tasks become increasingly automatic. Eventually we can learn to ride a bicycle 'with our eyes closed', as the saying goes. This is because the brain regions active in mediating an overlearned task (long-term procedural memory) are confined to subcortical regions alone, freeing up the cortex for more important system two-type work.

The retrieval of memories also appears to differ along procedural, semantic and episodic lines and between the intermediate and the long-term. Patients like H.M. who have suffered bilateral hippocampal damage experience *anterograde amnesia* (the inability to make new memories) both for specific events and for general facts. However, they can still learn new mechanical skills because procedural memory does not require the hippocampus. Additionally, amnesiacs tend to suffer *retrograde amnesia* (the inability to access memories made *before* the injury) going back several days, weeks, or sometimes years depending on the extent and severity of damage, again for semantic and episodic memories, but not for procedural skills. Because the hippocampus eventually transfers the memory traces into the cortex over many months to years, remote and childhood memories are paradoxically the last to go following traumatic amnesia or Alzheimer's dementia.

In summary, the hippocampus is required for intermediate and long-term encoding of semantic and episodic events and for intermediate recall of these events, but is not involved in long-term memory retrieval or in the processing of procedural memories. This means that there are separate systems for the encoding and retrieval of implicit, automatic, and mechanical skills on one hand, versus explicit conscious knowledge about the world and oneself on the other. The former relies preferentially on subcortical organs (the basal ganglia and cerebellum), while the latter requires the cortex and hippocampus.

As if things weren't complicated enough, the two types of explicit memories also appear to be stored in different parts of the brain. Functional MRI and *positron emission tomography* (PET) scan studies have demonstrated that the retrieval of episodic memories is associated with activity in the frontal and parietal lobes. Interestingly, the neuroscientist Endel Tulving has found that there is cortical asymmetry in the formation and access of personal memories. Imaging studies have revealed that the *left frontal lobe* is preferentially involved in *encoding* while the *right frontal lobe* is more active in *retrieval*. As a result, patients with isolated *right* frontal brain damage often suffer from profound retrograde amnesia for personal memories.

In contrast, semantic recall is associated with activation of the semantic space in the lateral temporal cortex. The hippocampus appears to be involved in both kinds of recall for recently acquired information (the name of the beautiful woman you met at the party last night, the word list you memorized for your spelling test), but not for remote recall of semantic information (name the seven continents). Remote autobiographical recall (what did you hate about kindergarten?) does, however, involve the hippocampus.

There seems to be something special about personal memories that has to do with the difference between *knowing* and *remembering*. The first involves the knowledge of something that exists independently of the observer, something that is objectively true regardless of whether or not you are around to question it. The other presumes the presence of a subject that possesses knowledge of something that it experienced in the past. The subjectivity inherent in the first-person account is necessarily dependent on an interpreter that creates and believes in the illusion of a coherent and continuous 'self'. This is the difference between semantic and episodic memory. The first is impersonal knowledge, the second is self-conscious recollection.

There is no shortage of theoretical models purporting to explain the functional anatomy of these two types of memory processing. Some notable scientists like Larry Squire think episodic memories are 'embedded' within semantic space, others like Endel Tulving believe that they are localized to different areas but that the retrieval of personal memories necessarily 'passes through' semantic memory. I shan't go into the nitty gritty, but suffice it to say that experimental evidence is somewhat inconclusive at this time. There are cases of patients, such as H.M., who have profound amnesia for personal memories with relatively intact semantic recall. In other words, they know more than they remember. On the other hand, there are as patients who suffer from severe agnosia for familiar objects, places, people (either names or faces), or facts in general, with intact autobiographical recall. These people remember more than they know. Knowing and remembering are two separate entities that are independent and dissociable.

The feeling or qualia of one's autobiographical memories may come from the frontal lobe and the limbic system, regions that are not active in semantic recall. The frontal cortex appears to imbue memories with a sense of personal intimacy. Patients with isolated damage to the frontal cortex, sparing the temporal lobes and the hippocampus, sometimes describe having strange recollections of events that they don't think they have actually experienced. Similar accounts come from patients following damage to the amygdala (more on this later). What they are describing is the loss of autonoetic consciousness, an awareness of oneself as the 'possessor' of a past experience. For them, personal memories are treated like just like semantic knowledge.

In the 1920's, the English psychologist Frederic Bartlett conducted studies on subjects' ability to recall the details of stories they had just read. He found that people invariably reconstruct a story in a more coherent and concise form, omitting or glossing over small details, while embellishing and reinterpreting what they took to be the main points. Moreover, as people were made to repeatedly retell the story from memory, more details tended to get lost while false elements were often grafted in. Eventually, the latest version from the multiple drafts of memory differed substantially from the original. Memory is, in a sense, much like perception: more a creative interpretation of external reality than an exact replica. Every time we recall an episode from our past, we are reconstructing not the initial event, but rather the last reconstruction of the previous reconstruction, and so on in a continuous regress. The hippocampus retrieval system indelibly stamps our present time and space information onto the target of our search with each recall command. The act of remembering necessarily alters the memory trace slightly so that we can never quite experience the past as it really was. What we are actually remembering is the memory of a memory of a memory… With each successive iteration, the contents become less faithful to the original because certain elements of our perceived present always creep into the process. After a time there might even be multiple separate versions of the same story competing for conscious attention. There is an unmistakable Darwinian aura to this whole process (replication, mutation, and selection), but let's leave this aside for now.

Let me make a brief comment on false memories. We have all experienced the feeling of having been somewhere or done something that never actually happened. These errors tend to crop up more frequently when we're fatigued, emotionally stressed, or in the midst of a novel situation, all of which tax the limited resources of our prefrontal executive system. The psychologist Elizabeth Loftus has done some compelling studies in which subjects were asked to recall specific incidents from their childhood. Loftus then altered some of these stories and then presented them back to the volunteers at a later time. Remarkably, a quarter of the subjects were convinced that the fabricated accounts were true. The facility with which people can be induced to believe false accounts by simply reminding them is especially disturbing in criminal cases, where the outcome often rests on eyewitness testimony. Young children are particularly prone to the power of suggestion. An expert prosecutor can easily get a frightened child to testify to all sorts of alleged abuse at the hands of a completely innocent defendant.

An individual may not be able to distinguish between a true and false memory, but neuroscientists armed with the latest brain scanner often can. True recall of episodic information activates the hippocampus, temporal cortex, and the right dorsilateral PFC. False recall involves these areas plus the orbitofrontal PFC as well. It appears that making up something that never happened requires more mental effort than remembering something that did. Recall from the last chapter that the DLPFC is the locus for working memory while the OFC is important for emotional integration. These two prefrontal areas work together to construct the most coherent and meaningful possible account based on a true story, but certain characters and events may be altered and details may be embellished for the enjoyment of the audience. An intact and mature PFC is necessary to distinguish truth from fiction. This is why children, and patients suffering from dementia, alcoholic psychosis, and traumatic brain damage are so prone to confabulate.

Prodigy
The editor of one's autobiography is the left hemisphere interpreter. But what if we could somehow turn off the interpreter? Would false accounts disappear? Would episodic memories become crystal clear? Would knowledge hitherto buried in the recesses of the subconscious suddenly become near and dear? These are intriguing possibilities that clearly need more research funding. The storage capacity of the brain is not infinite, but it is a whole lot bigger than what most of us use on a day-to-day basis. We can begin to appreciate this by examining cases of extraordinarily enhanced memory, the savants.

Some of the mental feats associated with savant syndrome are so stunning as to appear supernatural. A young Englishman named Daniel Tammet, as documented in the wonderful BBC documentary Brainman, learned Icelandic in a week and memorized pi to 22,514 decimal places. Not to be outdone, the Japanese prodigy Hideaki Tomoyori raised the bar to 40,000 digits. Kim Peek, an autistic savant who was the inspiration for the movie, 'Rainman', is said to have memorized every page of every book he has ever read (currently over 10,000 including the Encyclopaedia Britannica, Shakespeare's complete works, the Oxford English Dictionary, and the King James Bible). The German mathematical prodigy R. Gamm can calculate the cube root of any six-digit number to nine decimal places in his head and tell if a seven-digit number is a prime within a few seconds. The English autistic artist Stephen Wiltshire, popularized by Oliver Sacks in <u>An Anthropologist on Mars</u>, can memorize a building or urban landscape in a few minutes and sketch it in photographic detail from memory years later. The Russian psychologist Alexander Luria described the case of Shereshevskii, a man with a memory so prodigious that he was unable to forget anything that ever happened to him. In fact, he was said to have been tortured by his incessantly recurring memories.

There is, of course, nothing supernatural about these remarkable minds. Their brains are made of neurons, synapses, neurotransmitters, and genes that look and work just like those of everyone else. What is special is the way they use their various neural modules in combination when solving problems and perceiving the world. Autistic people are known to pay more attention to minute details such as crosshatch patterns on a carpet or background noise than on the global picture. While most autistics are not savants, most savants are far along on the autistic spectrum. So it is not surprising that savant skills are generally limited to rote memorization and lightning calculation than to anything that requires much analysis or deep insight. Normal people certainly have the same neural substrate as savants, but the innate drive for central coherence seems to inhibit lower level processing from reaching consciousness. Whether this inhibition is hardwired from birth or acquired through early childhood experience is unknown. It the latter is true, it opens up the tantalizing possibility that these amazing savant skills may somehow be 'unmasked' in ordinary people.

Another point of difference between the neurotypical and the savant brain is the knack for warping sensory processing across multiple modalities, such as sights and sounds. This ability is called synesthesia, and it is much more common in savants than in the general population. Daniel Temmet, for instance, claims that numbers have distinctive three-dimensional shapes, colors, and 'personalities' which make them stand out. His pi memorization was made much easier because it had a specific 'landscape' in his mind's eye. All he had to do was visualize this landscape and the numbers simply revealed themselves. This seems plausible in terms of memorization technique, but it is more difficult to explain his ability to do lightning fast arithmetic. When asked how he can multiply two random eight-digit numbers within a few seconds, Temmet claimed that he doesn't actually do any mental calculation at all, but that the solution is simply there in visual form in some obscure corner of his mental space to which he can navigate.

Savant skills and memories have a naturalness about them that is uncontaminated by the interpretative mechanism. This is very different from normally learned skills, which require conscious effort. We recognize that our ability to learn a foreign language or do arithmetic in our heads is a creative process. Once learned, they become part of us. There is an intimate relationship between our skills, knowledge, and memories and our sense of personal identity. We become what we know. The savant ability to calculate cube roots, recite pi, perceive perfect pitch, or paint a landscape from memory are more semantic than autobiographical; they may be pure but are strangely dissociated from their personalities.

From Knowledge to Belief
And you may find yourself in a beautiful house, with a beautiful wife.
And you may ask yourself – well…how did I get here?
And you may tell yourself
This is not my beautiful house!
And you may tell yourself
This is not my beautiful wife!

Talking Heads

Is it possible to know something without believing it or believe something without knowing it? There is an exceedingly curious disorder that sheds some light on this distinction. The annals of neurology and psychiatry make occasional references to patients who, usually following a blow to the head, begin to insist that their loved ones are not really who they seem to be. Mothers, fathers, wives, husbands, children, and sometimes even pet dogs and cats may look and act like the ones they once knew so well, but that feeling of familiarity has somehow gone away. Tormented by their confusion, these patients eventually conclude that these exemplars are just 'impostors' masquerading as the real thing. This remarkable delusion is called *Capgras' syndrome.*

Capgras' patients are not demented, amnesic, or perceptually impaired. Their intelligence, semantic knowledge, and episodic memory (mediated by the hippocampus and the temporal cortex) are preserved. Their ability to perceive faces (through the fusiform face area) is intact, as is their ability to express and feel emotion (via the amygdala). They have no delusions that strangers, casual acquaintances, or landmarks are replaced by replicas. And intriguingly, the loved ones who look to them like impostors sound 'real' when only their voices are heard on the phone. What in heaven's name is going on here? The answer comes not from God, but from neuroscience.

What appears to be going on in Capgras' delusion is that there is a disconnection between the amygdala and the fusiform face region. Normally, when one looks at a person's face, the visual information is processed through the ventral stream to its termination in the fusiform gyrus. Damage to these areas produces agnosia (the inability to perceive shapes) and prosopagnosia (the failure to recognize faces), respectively. Many of the neurons in the fusiform area send axon fibers deep into the semantic space of the temporal cortex where the repository of familiar faces is stored. When you see your child, your brain first processes the features of her face and then searches its memory bank for a match. The near simultaneous activity in the fusiform/temporal region marks the intersection between perception and memory. The same thing happens when you see anything else that is familiar. But perception is also linked strongly to emotion.

In addition to the temporal cortex, the fusiform gyrus is connected to the amygdala, the gateway to the limbic system. Bilateral damage to the amygdala itself causes the inability to feel and express emotions. But a disconnection in the wires linking face perception to the amygdala causes something quite different. Recall that dopamine neurons in the limbic system imbue certain perceptions and memories with saliency and anticipation. The things and events that have affected our lives, positively or negatively, are stored in our memory bank with an emotional tag made of dopamine. Whenever we relive or recollect those things that are emotionally salient, their perception and/or memory triggers the amygdala all over again, and the feelings of love or hate, dread or excitement, as the case may be, come rushing forth automatically. In the case of faces, an intact circuit from the fusiform area to the amydala on both sides of the brain is necessary. When this circuit is up and running, a face that we have learned to associate with good memories (your newborn baby daughter's, for instance) activates the amygdala's connections to the autonomic nervous system (via the hypothalamus), the endocrine system (via the hypothalamic/pituitary axis), and the prefrontal cortex. The result is that your entire body, not just your brain, responds to the sight of your loved one with a quickened pulse and a warm tingling in your palms. These signals are then picked up by the brain allowing you to feel the emotion of love. And if you are fortunate enough to reach out and touch your loved one, the tactile information stimulates a rush of oxytocin from the posterior pituitary that simultaneously dampens the amygdala and makes you feel drawn in even further. This is what love is. Unfortunately, those suffering from Capgras' syndrome cannot feel any of it.

Think about it this way: semantic space sends multiple parallel channels to the amygdala. Each channel represents some aspect of your memory that can elicit an emotion. When any of these channels are blocked off, you no longer feel the emotion of a particular memory. Capgras' syndrome is just one particular case, albeit a dramatic one, of a blockage between memory/perception and emotion. But faces are not the only things stored in our knowledge banks. Countless animals, buildings, foods, places, events, stories, customs, and, in fact, any concept which can be learned and discerned have access to the limbic system, and any of them can be selectively cut off. Cutting a wire makes the subject it represented emotionally unfamiliar. An intriguing possibility is that perhaps millions of otherwise normal people who are described as emotionally distant may have milder subclinical forms of Capgras as a result of congenitally weaker connections to the amygdala.

A final point worth making is that the amygdala appears to have a cognitive function quite apart from its role in emotion. We have seen how its neurons label salient stimuli with physiological reactions (emotions), but they also label them with a sense of general familiarity. In the course of human evolution, those ancestors who were better able to catagorize things in the world as dangerous or desirable had a significant survival advantage over those who could not. Life becomes a whole lot easier, and sometimes safer, when one is able to get the gist or feel for something early on without having to verify every novel detail. I believe that the ability to stereotype situations or people in this way arose in the limbic system.

Capgras' patients have been known to make errors on tests of categorization, for example, being able to tell if several photographs taken from different angles are of the same building or person. Normal subjects are very good at distilling the important characteristics of an object or situation so that they get a general sense of what it is regardless of how it was seen or experienced. You know that a particular church is the same church in the morning's light or the evening's gloaming or under a brilliant cover of snow. You know that the little girl in that grainy picture is your mother even as you acknowledge her as the frail old woman in front of you right now. But is she really the same person? Your temporal lobe, and basic physics, would tell you no. It is not just appearances that change with time; memories and molecules do too. None of the atoms that made up your mother all those years ago are in her body now. The thoughts in her head now are not the thoughts she had then. And yet we know, we feel, and we believe, that they share a common essence. The ventral stream and semantic space are good at telling similar looking things apart. The amygdala is good at telling what dissimilar looking things have in common. The ability to generalize is not limited to the limbic system; the prefrontal cortex can do this too. But it is in the limbic system that the appreciation of the essence of something is coupled to the expression and feeling of emotion that it engenders. Essence is what makes things 'real' to us. It also gives us a sense of a continuously existing self. Out of this convergence comes belief.

One wonders whether those with Capgras' syndrome can even appreciate the very concept of self: a self that endures in space and time and maintains its identity despite continuous assaults on its physical, biological, and psychological integrity. If these people cannot distill the underlying essences of themselves or of the ones they love, then how can they possibly love them or even believe in them as anything other than passing sensations or transient activations of semantic space?

We can look at this schematically (Figure 9). Information flows from perception to memory to emotion. Damage to perceptual areas causes any of a number of agnosias. Damage to memory areas causes any of a number of amnesias. Agnosias and amnesias are diseases of too little knowledge. On the other hand, hypertrophy of perception and/or memory can lead to the savant syndrome, which is a disease of too much knowledge. Damage to the connections between the memory areas and the emotional areas causes Capgras' syndrome, which is a disease of emotional blindness and too little belief. But what if there is hypertrophy of the connections to the emotional areas? Would we end up with a disease of too much emotional vision and belief? The answer again lies in the annals of neurology.

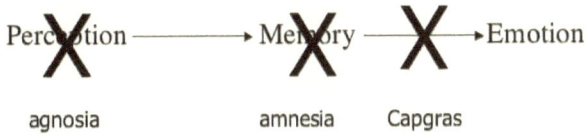

Figure 9

The God Module

Just as truth, knowledge, and memory are distinct, so too are knowledge and belief dissociable. Capgras' delusions are examples of knowledge without belief. But is it possible to have belief without knowledge? Over the last two decades, the stimulant drug methylenedioxymethamphetamine (MDMA), better known by its street name, Ecstasy, has become ubiquitous in the youth rave scene worldwide. Teenage partygoers claim that the drug mellows them out, gets rid of their anxieties, and makes them feel more connected to the people around them (usually other Ecstasy-popping strangers freaking out on the dance floor). Ecstasy works by dumping all the stored-up serotonin, dopamine, and norepinephrine into the synapses of the central nervous system, effectively stimulating all mental processes for a few hours before the inevitable crash. Researchers have found that in addition to the euphoria associated with other stimulants like cocaine and nicotine, Ecstasy also produces a sense of intimacy, empathy, insight, heightened senses, and short-term amnesia. For these reasons, the drug enjoyed a brief period of popularity, before the FDA banned it, among some psychotherapists treating patients with severe anxiety and post-traumatic stress disorder.

What is interesting about Ecstasy is the association of its trademark euphoric effect with the feeling of enlightenment on the one hand and amnesia on the other. It is as if there are three intersecting dimensions of happiness, belief, and memory (Figure 10). The release of serotonin and dopamine produces an increase in happiness and belief respectively, but not in memory. Memory is more dependent on another neurotransmitter called glutamate, and its receptor, NMDA. Of course, this is a grossly simplified model of much more complex, dynamic, and messy processes in the brain. These things cannot be reduced to just three unknown variables. But I think it is an instructive way to begin to think about how the physical brain enables the mind to construct belief systems independently of memory and knowledge.

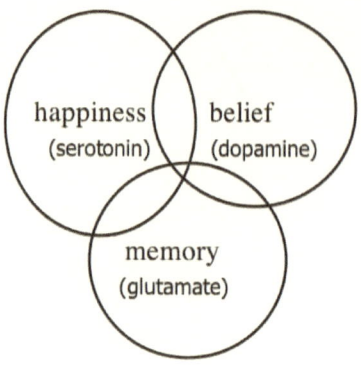

Figure 10

There is a deliciously bizarre disorder in the psychoanalytical literature that is in some ways a mirror image of Capgras' syndrome. Fregoli delusion is characterized by the persistent belief that random strangers are really familiar people in disguise. Moreover, they believe that these characters are out to get them. Delusions of persecution and false attributions of significance to random people and events are usually linked to psychotic states like paranoid schizophrenia. But who among us has never mistaken a stranger for someone we know? This tends to happen more often when we're thinking about someone dear who can't be with us at the moment. We seek them so desperately that our brains trick us into 'seeing' them in everyone. I suspect that our overcharged limbic systems fire a top-down modulation signal on our visual cortex powerful enough to bias incoming sensory information. We see only what we want to see, and become blinkered to everything else.

In full-blown Fregoli syndrome, however, the delusion becomes negative and persecutory. The explanation for this might be too many connections between the amygdala – the source of fear and anxiety – and the fusiform face area. Whenever a Fregoli patient sees a face, familiar or otherwise, her amygdala automatically pushes the panic button. The fight or flight response is nonspecific, but the interpreter demands an explanation. So it adroitly splices a specific rationale into the story: 'that stranger staring at me right now is really that damn traffic cop who ticketed me last week.' Speculation aside, it seems reasonable to say that belief, like memory, comes from a blending of perception and interpretation. The perception may actually be closer to reality than the interpretation is, but it is the interpretation that we come to believe.

This brings us to the temporal lobe. If there is one part of the brain where religion happens, this is it. There are two compelling reasons. First is the neuroanatomy. All those players I described earlier as being important for knowledge, memory, emotion, and belief are found here. The ventral stream, the fusiform face area, semantic space, the hippocampus, the hypothalamus, and the amygdala are all crammed into the confines of the temporal lobe. Second is the characteristic 'religious personality' associated with temporal lobe epilepsy.

Temporal lobe epilepsy or TLE is a disorder characterized by abnormal neurological activity (seizures) arising from somewhere in the temporal lobe, such as the amygdala, hippocampus, or, less commonly, the cortex itself. TLE can be caused by brain tumors, trauma, infections, abnormal blood vessels, or occasionally, a genetic mutation, but for a large proportion of patients, no cause can be found. Epileptic seizures usually start from one focal part of the brain and either stay there or spread outwards over a period of several seconds. If the seizure ultimately crosses the corpus callosum to involve the opposite hemisphere, the patient has a classic grand mal seizure involving generalized convulsions and loss of consciousness. These are medical emergencies requiring prompt treatment with anticonvulsant medications. But if it remains localized to the area around the focus (simple partial seizures), much more interesting things can happen.

It has been recognized for some time that individuals afflicted with simple partial seizures of their temporal lobe often report very peculiar experiences. They include auditory or olfactory hallucinations, the recall of long lost memories (or the loss of well remembered ones), an eerie sense of having experienced a situation before (déjà vu), or an equally weird feeling of unfamiliarity with an otherwise well known situation (jamais vu). Fregoli and Capgras' syndromes, which are in some sense analogous to déjà vu and jamais vu respectively, have also been found to co-segregate with TLE. A subset of TLE patients becomes hyper-religious. These colorful characters walk around claiming to have found God, or the cosmic significance of all things, or the meaning of life, or some other such nonsense.

Chronic hyper-religiosity in the setting of TLE is different from the acute hallucinations and amnesias sometimes associated with the seizure activity itself. These people believe in their newfound faith even when they're not having seizures. Psychiatrists sometimes call this the 'temporal lobe personality'. It is as if the religious hallucination produced by each seizure leaves an afterglow that eventually alters the personality permanently. Many famous people are said to have suffered from temporal lobe personality syndrome, including Moses, Isaiah, Jesus, Mohammad, the Buddha, and the writers Fyodor Dostoevsky, Lewis Carroll, Phillip K. Dick, and Sylvia Plath. These cannot be proved, unfortunately, as their brains are no longer available for pathologists to dissect. They may just as well have suffered from schizophrenia, bipolar disorder, narcissistic personality trait, or some combination of the above. But the possibility remains very intriguing indeed.

Why do many people with temporal lobe seizures become hyper-religious? What is the connection between the temporal lobe and belief in general? It all comes back to the connections between the limbic system and semantic space. I think what's happening is that the amygdala, in response to something perceived, remembered, or imagined, extracts the essence of whatever is currently held in attention and generates an emotional response to it. This is the critical neural correlate for religious belief: when whatever is activated in semantic space becomes imbued with emotional gist. The semantic or episodic knowledge initially triggers the limbic system, but the resulting noise of the belief engine soon drowns it out. Belief is a pearl. Underneath multiple layers of illusory opulence, there lies a kernel of knowledge. But the objectivity of that knowledge is blurred by our natural tendency to generalize and reframe it in the context of our subjective emotional responses.

Is the illusion of enlightenment limited to patients afflicted with TLE? The answer is a resounding no. Billions of 'normal' people profess to a belief in the existence of supernatural forces, and a large proportion of them claim to have experienced these forces personally. They cannot all be suffering from seizures or Fregoli syndrome or an Ecstasy overdose. Clearly, temporal lobe/amygdala hyper-connectivity happens to the majority of human beings at least some of the time. And there is evidence that it can be induced artificially. Canadian psychologist Michael Persinger conducted an experiment in which he stimulated his own temporal lobes with a device called a trans-cranial magnetic stimulator (TMS). When held up to the head, the machine discharges a powerful magnetic field to the underlying brain, in effect creating a simulated seizure. Persinger, a self-professed atheist, reported that he experienced God for the first time in his life when he put on his 'God helmet'. Perhaps his experience was really no different from what Buddhist monks, Hindu yogis, and new age mystics feel when they reach a deep state of meditation. All their paths converge on the magical belief center of their limbic systems.

The neuroscientist V.S. Ramachandran has conducted some interesting experiments on hyper-religious TLE patients. He showed them a series of words or pictures while they were hooked up to a galvanic skin sensor, a machine that measures the amount of electrical resistance from their sweaty palms, which in turn is a pretty good indicator of one's anxiety level. Incidentally, the galvanic skin response, or GSR, is the basis for the lie detector test. The images were of religious nature (crosses or churches), violence (scenes of auto wrecks or dead bodies), sex (pornographic centerfolds), or neutral (pictures of shoes, tables, and so on). Most people normally demonstrate an increased GSR when viewing sexual or violent themes compared to the religious or neutral ones. But the TLE patients exhibited a markedly increased GSR when shown religious images but an abnormally reduced GSR in association with the violent or sexual images. Ramachandran interpreted this finding as evidence that hyper-religious TLE patients may have an enhanced neural circuit that specifically codes for religious experience.

I want to emphasize here that religious experience is not a place, but rather a physical and biochemical process that happens in the brain. If you dissect the temporal cortex or the amygdala of a monkey or a human being, you will not find God. You can magnify a frozen tissue section 10,000 times with an electron microscope, fix it with special stains or antibodies, or hybridize it to RNA probes, and what you will find is a bewildering jungle of neurons, axon fibers, synapses, and molecules, but again, no God. These are just static snapshots. Yet, the temporal lobe is precisely where our experience of God happens. The trick is that the process of magical thought requires many other regions of a healthy brain working dynamically together, within a community of other interacting brains, all wrapped up in a cultural milieu. But a new technique called multielectrode recording that involves inserting tiny electrodes inside a living conscious temporal lobe (preferably of a TLE patient undergoing brain surgery), may potentially give us a 'moving picture' of the religious process. Stay tuned.

Baby Brains
We now know where religion is in the brain, but what exactly is it, and how did it get there? Since the magical thoughts that constitute religion are pervasive throughout human cultures, one can make the assumption that there is an innate religious instinct built into our brains. This assumption is fraught as plenty of people (including a surprising number of academics) still stubbornly refuse to accept that anything in our minds is innate despite the mounting evidence. So to approach this question, it would be instructive to examine how mental faculties in general develop in healthy human brains, and extrapolate to religious belief from there. Child psychologists have already carried out quite a lot of fascinating research in this department.

Babies are born into this world helpless and ignorant, but they're not stupid. They have amazing intuitions about the physical, biological, mechanical, and psychological worlds around them. The problem is that infants are not very good at telling us what's going on in their minds. The psychologists Elizabeth Spelke and Renée Baillargeon developed a way to get around this by gauging the length of time infants spent staring at objects on a video screen. If something surprising captured their attention, their brains needed time to process it; if they got bored, they looked somewhere else. Using stare time as a measuring stick, the researchers conducted a series of experiments designed to probe how much babies know about physical concepts. They found that infants stared longer when shown that two sticks that moved together behind a partially occluding screen turned out to be separate sticks when the screen was removed, than if they turned out to be parts of the same object. They stared longer when a billiard ball started to move before it was struck by another ball, than when it moved after it was struck. They demonstrated long stare times when an object that passed behind a screen was revealed to have morphed into two objects or disappeared completely. These experiments prove that babies as young as four months of age, long before they have a chance to flunk their physics classes, already have an intuitive grasp of object permanence, continuity, momentum, and causation. Psychologists call this folk physics, and it is part of the innate mental toolkit with which all of us are born.

But wait, there's more. Three and four-year olds appreciate the difference between living and nonliving things. If you show a preschool child a video of a coffeepot and then convert it into something else, such as a makeshift birdfeeder, the child will tell you that the coffeepot is now a birdfeeder. But if you show them a porcupine and morph it into a hairbrush or a cactus, they won't tell you that it's now a hairbrush. They'll say it's a funny looking porcupine. Psychologists who have conducted experiments like these have concluded that children are innate believers of essentialism, the notion that an object can possess an inherent essence quite independent of its external appearance. And they apply essentialism to living things, but not to inanimate objects. Children are vague when asked what this essence is exactly. They may say it's the 'thing that makes them what they are', for instance. Adults are also natural believers of essentialism, and it explains why the genetic theory of inheritance had such a hard time overcoming the old myth of 'vitalism' to which some people still cling. Like intuitive physics, folk biology is something that develops independently of parents and teachers.

The separation of biology from physics in the mind is something our brains are simply hardwired to do. The cognitive machinery has a modular design made up of many different domain-specific knowledge systems, each of them taking up a particular part of the cortex. We have seen some of them already, including the face-processing system in the fusiform gyrus. Living things occupy another area of the temporal lobe's semantic space.

And this space is probably subdivided into modules specializing in plants versus animals. The animal space may be further subdivided into predator versus prey versus competitor, and so on down the taxonomic ladder. Other modules perhaps located in the motor areas of the frontal and parietal lobes handle folk physics.

Non-living things are also organized according to category. Natural objects such as rocks and clouds are processed by different brain areas than man-made artifacts such as tools and automobiles. Both kinds of objects activate semantic space in the lateral temporal lobe, but artifacts also light up the premotor areas of the parietal lobe. Children as young as eighteen months have an intuitive understanding that tools like hammers and forks have to be handled in a specific way as opposed to random pieces of plastic. Give a novel tool-like object to any kid old enough to speak, and he will ask you what it's for. Solid evidence for this dissociation comes from cases of brain damage that affects a person's knowledge of how to use an artifact (motor apraxia), but not her ability to identify it (agnosia), and vice versa. The knowledge of tools requires the understanding of function, which is something quite distinct from the appreciation of form. And function implies purpose, design, and intention.

Agency and the Theory of Mind

The divisions of things into living versus inanimate or natural versus manmade are just two of the ways the mind parses reality. Another is by apparent behavior. Most entities (natural kinds like rocks, water, or projectiles) simply follow the rules of folk physics. Other things, such as animals and some self-propelled machines, seem to possess an internal drive that predictably pushes them towards a goal (food, females, or a patch of dust) that would be very unlikely to happen by chance. And yet a third group of things behaves erratically, changing its goals depending on situation or mood. Dan Dennett calls them the physical, design, and intentional stances, respectively. These are three separate cognitive interpretations of the physical world of molecules and forces in terms of macroscopic bodies, goal-directed agents, or individuals possessed of free will.

Babies can normally discriminate among the three stances quite early on. We have already discussed their facility with intuitive physics and man-made artifacts. By the age of twelve months, they begin to interpret cartoons of bouncing dots and moving geometrical figures as agents with specific desires. For example, babies who've seen a dot 'jump over' an obstruction on its way to another dot expect it to make a beeline to its companion in the absence of the obstruction. They express surprise, in terms of increased stare time, if the dot jumps over a nonexistent wall. By three years of age, when children are able to talk, they will invariably explain the same cartoon with a story of the dot 'wanting to' get close to its companion. Most, but not all, children get this concept naturally. Autistic children do not. This is because there is an innate agency detection device in the brain that is normally genetically programmed to go on-line between one to two years of age.

The agent detector device (ADD) is a cognitive module that allows its user to recognize any object that might have a mind of its own. Like other inference systems such as motion detectors, face detectors, predator detectors, and object describers, it is hardwired to the sense organs, the motor centers, the limbic system, and semantic space to give fast and automatic responses. Moreover, these modules are also hooked up to each other. It seems likely that the ADD works by integrating input from the parts of the brain specializing in the perception of biological motion, eye movement (gaze direction), and facial expression. It is easy to see how the information in these combined channels can build up a coherent picture of a free agent. Something that looks and acts alive, expresses emotion, and directs its gaze at a target may be something worth paying attention to.

The ADD is the foundation for a more complex mental organ that allows humans to understand what other agents might be thinking about. This is the so-called 'Theory of Mind Module' (TOMM), first coined by a trio of English psychologists specializing in autism research: Uta Frith, Simon Baron-Cohen, and Alan Leslie. Theory of mind (TOM) itself is an older concept that goes back to the work of Dan Dennett and the anthropologist Dan Sperber. The thinking goes like this. Different people have different mental states. Is it possible that one person might know or believe something that a second person does not? The core idea of TOM is that knowledge and belief are relative. It is the ability to attribute a particular mental state or point-of-view that is not one's own to another agent. Having a TOMM enables one to appreciate the fact that others may have false beliefs, which, in turn, makes deception, duplicity, lying, and cheating possible.

Mind reading begins as early as age two. Children of this age normally start to engage in pretend play. By age four, children regularly practice the art of deception. Most of them will also pass simple TOM tests. In other words, they understand when someone has a false belief. Most autistic kids never pass this test at any age. Autism is therefore a perfect natural experiment for investigating the implications of TOM and its absence. Those on the autism spectrum fail to develop a working TOMM (they also may or may not have a defective ADD, depending on severity), and hence suffer from what Simon Baron-Cohen calls 'mindblindness'. As a result, they cannot grasp the fact that others may not know or believe or feel the same things they do. And inversely, they have a difficult time understanding what others may know, believe, or feel unless they're explicitly told. Autistics are notoriously gullible and easily manipulated; on the other hand, they are wonderfully honest and straightforward in their own self-centered way.

I believe that the TOMM lies inside the domain of a dedicated ADD. It is possible for one to have the ability to detect an agent and respond appropriately to it (fight or flee or feed or copulate) without knowing that it has its own beliefs. In fact, the TOMM probably arose out of an ADD in the course of evolution. But the converse is not true. The talent for perceiving agency and intention is necessary but not sufficient for theory of mind. Intuitive psychology requires another crucial component: recursive logic.

Language and Recursive Logic
The linguistic philosopher Ray Jackendorf has pointed out an interesting commonality in rather ordinary sentences like these:

> The messenger *went from* Paris *to* Istanbul.
> The inheritance finally *went to* Fred.
> The light *went from* green *to* red.
> The meeting *went from* 3:00 *to* 4:00.

All of the sentences above indicate a change of location. Yet only in the first example is there any physical movement. The other three describe a shift of possession, a change of state, and a change in time. Although nothing actually moves from location A to location B, we speak as if they do. The fact that statements like these sound so natural to us supports the notion that human beings have an innate tendency to think *metaphorically*. Ample evidence for this comes from studies of children, who spontaneously coin their own metaphors for desire, intention, and belief using the language of physical action.

Here are some examples from preschool children collected by the psychologist Melissa Bowerman [Pinker, Steven How the Mind Works, pages 356-357]:

> You put me just bread and butter.
> Mother takes ball away from boy and puts it to girl.

> I'm taking these cracks bigger [while shelling a peanut].
> I putted part of the sleeve blue so I crossed it out with red [while coloring].

> Can I have any reading behind the dinner?

Today we'll be packing because tomorrow there won't be enough space to pack.

Friday is covering Saturday and Sunday so I can't have Saturday and Sunday if I don't go through Friday.

My dolly is scrunched from someone…but not from me.
They had to stop from a red light.

Linguists have collected thousands of similar metaphors from every language ever studied. Such metaphorical representations of intentions are, to excuse the expression, built 'on top of' ideas about actions. See what I mean? This makes quite a lot of sense in terms of evolutionary psychology. Animals, including humans, must constantly evaluate and negotiate their physical surroundings by calculating distance (to the nearest waterhole, fertile female, hiding place) and force (to crack a nut, break a branch, push the bad guy off a cliff). We know that there are discrete brain regions designed to accomplish these things – the dorsal visual system and the premotor cortex, respectively. We also know that natural selection does not create structures and modules from scratch. Body parts used for one purpose (fins for swimming, jaw bones for chewing) become co-opted for other functions in descendent species (limbs for crawling, middle ear bones for hearing). An analogous process may have occurred in our ancestral primate brain – giving rise to a 'metaphor representation module' for understanding social action from a vestigial 'action perception module' for understanding physical causality. While it is still important for humans to understand and manipulate inanimate objects and calculate projectile trajectories, it is arguably even more important to understand and manipulate other people and calculate social decisions, because we are essentially evolved social animals. We view all aspects of our social lives through the filter of intention. If we could somehow remove that filter, the world would seem a truly strange place; a place without free will or responsibility: a world of funny looking automatons wandering aimlessly.

What is the nature of this innate metaphor representation system and how is it related to TOM? The psychologist Alan Leslie has proposed the idea of a 'decoupler'. This is a dedicated brain module that transforms knowledge of the physical world into a proposition between subject and object. For instance, a mother holding a banana to her ear can be decoupled into the metarepresentation, "the mother pretends the banana is a telephone." The agent (the mother) possesses an attitude (pretends-true) towards the thought content (is a telephone) referring to another object (banana). This mental grammar is highly versatile at representing all sorts of intentional stances that people may take: [a] [believes/does not believe/desires/does not desire] that [x] is [true/false y, etc]. It is flexible enough to be used in recursive loops: 'I believe that she thought that it was false...'

The decoupler allows one to represent another's representation of something even if one knows that the second representation is in error: 'Ptolemy thought that the sun and planets revolved around the earth.' The embedding of one representation into another (*metarepresentation*) is the essence of first-order TOM. This can be elaborated into second, third, fourth, or even higher-order TOM: 'Copernicus thought that Ptolemy thought that the sun and planets revolved around the earth.' Decoupling belief states from reality lies at the core of social and cultural understanding. Without it, one could not appreciate sarcasm, satire, irony, wit; one would read novels, but miss the stuff 'between the lines'; listen to jokes, but miss the punchline. The person without a decoupler would lack imagination and creativity.

Metarepresentation is a type of recursive logic essential not just for TOM, but also for language and mathematics, which also use embedded structures. For example, $a^2-b^2=(a-b)(a+b)$. The linguistic and mathematical fluency of some higher functioning autistics who nonetheless fail simple Theory of Mind tests indicates that recursive logic, while necessary for all three abilities, is not sufficient for TOM (Figure 11). I believe that innate language, mathematics, and TOM all require a recursion module, but that TOM also requires an independent ADD.

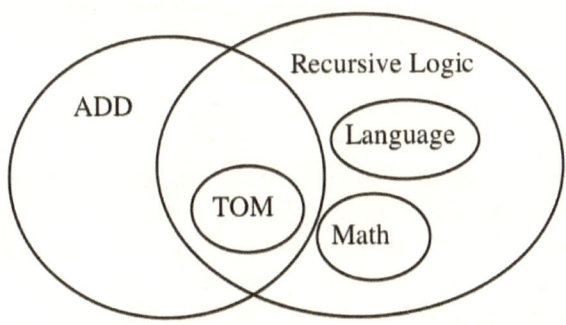

Figure 11

Universal Grammar

The ability to communicate via language, whether written, spoken, or sign, distinguishes humans from just about all other animals. We don't know how language evolved since gestures and voices don't fossilize. Written records can take us back several thousand years, but speech was already well established by then. The psychologist Michael Corballis proposes that spoken language developed from a form of sign language some 100,000 years ago, corresponding to the last great human migration out of Africa [see Corballis, <u>From Hand to Mouth: the Origins of Language</u>, 2002]. But his theory assumes that proto-language in the form of symbolic gestures already existed long before we started to talk. We need to start by examining the behavior of the great majority of living things on earth that has no language at all.

Communication between individuals in the animal kingdom has evolved amazing complexity. Bumblebee dances, birdcalls, and whale songs all involve intricate coordination of muscles to produce stereotyped messages for the benefit of others. Through them, other bees find the source of food, birds defend their territory, and orphan orcas find their pods thousands of miles away. Some animals, such as the vervet monkey, have even mastered symbolic representation.

There are two features of human communication that make it unique in the animal kingdom. First is the attribution of meaning to otherwise arbitrary actions such as a finger flick, a hum, a click, or a high-pitched shriek. Very few animals are capable of this. The second is the recombination of these meaningful units (words and word stems) in a linear sequence in time (phrases and sentences) to depict thoughts, stories, and desires. This double combinatorial system of sounds/gestures into meaning, and then meaning into stories is known as the *duality of patterning*. As any student of elementary math knows, combinatorial systems generate an endless variety of possibilities from a limited number of building blocks. A finite number of hand and facial gestures, sounds, or letters of the alphabet can be used to generate a very large number of possible words, each with a slightly different meaning. This is known as *semantics*. Additionally, a limited number of words (roughly 20,000 per language, but over 100,000 for Standard English, not counting further hundreds of thousands of scientific and technical terms) can be used to generate a near infinite number of possible sentences, each expressing a different story. It is the second type of patterning, from meaningful units (words) to sentences, that is uniquely human. This is grammar.

Grammar, or *syntax*, is the way bits of meaning are combined to become coherent for those with whom one is communicating. Contrary to what one may believe, the basic rules of grammar are not the product of some arbitrary cultural convention. They are hardwired into every normal child's brain. Children are not born talking, but by age two they start constructing single words out of meaningless babble. By two and a half, they start combining words into simple sentences. By age three, their language development literally explodes into a non-stop riot of exclamations, exhortations, inquiries, and imperatives, many of which are, quite unintentionally, profoundly humorous or humorously profound. No matter what the mother tongue or the native culture may be, the unfolding of the linguistic developmental timetable is constant for every child on earth.

There is universality not only in the childhood acquisition of the language instinct, but also within language itself. The basic components of the sentence: subject, verb, and object in English (or subject, object, followed by verb in most other languages), are used by all children in all cultures whether or not they learn them in school. Those annoying language-specific details such as gender, irregular conjugation, and odd plural forms must, of course, be learned, along with the vast lexicon (vocabulary). This is what parents, teachers, and television are for. But the rules of basic grammar naturally unfold in a specific sequence in the course of normal child development.

If there is a fundamental grammar independent of learning, culture, or mother tongue, how and when did it come about? Let me make two points: first, no animals, not even dolphins, chimpanzees, or parrots, have any natural grammar. They may be undoubtedly clever, emotional creatures with good memories, the ability to learn faces and signs, and perhaps solve a few simple problems using symbolic logic. But we have no evidence that they use a combinatorial system of syntax. Even with painstaking training, chimps are only able to master a few rules of grammar. And it seems likely that they learn them by memorization of particular examples rather than through generalization. Since chimps are our closest surviving cousins on the evolutionary tree, we can be fairly certain that grammar evolved sometime after our common ancestral line diverged about seven million years ago in the Great Rift Valley.

Second, grammar is not limited to speech. Deaf people learn to communicate in 'grammatical' sign language. Deaf children raised in the absence of formal sign language, but in proximity to other deaf peers, spontaneously invent their own gestural language. Such languages have their own syntactic organization, somewhat akin to the unconventional grammar of Creole languages, which develop from the talk of illiterate children of polyglot 'pidgin' speaking parents. Thus, grammar is not limited to speaking people with a literate background.

Then there are those rare people who never develop grammar. Those born with a disorder called *Specific Language Impairment*, which I will describe in more detail later, are otherwise intelligent people with a mutated 'grammar gene'. People suffering strokes to the left prefrontal region known as *Broca's area* usually lose the ability to speak and write grammatically, although their thoughts may be largely unimpaired. Finally, there are reports of unfortunate children who for one reason or another were socially isolated for the first few years of life and grow up to be partially or sometimes even totally incapable of grammatical speech. These observations indicate that the language instinct is independent of speech, localized to fairly specific parts of the brain, largely genetic, and relatively recently evolved. In addition, it is an instinct that requires the proper social environment to come on line.

Syntax gradually evolved over thousands of generations as numerous genes involved in brain growth and differentiation accumulated random mutations. It almost certainly didn't happen overnight as a result of one mega-mutation, or a 'Eureka!' moment of insight by some long forgotten caveman genius. Theories abound as to how and why syntax actually evolved. One explanation is that it's simply a function of increasing brain size and general intelligence. But that can't be right because grammar is too modular and specialized to have just happened once we attained sufficient brain mass. It is also quite dissociable from general intelligence (there are smart people who can't communicate and good communicators who aren't very smart).

Another group of hypotheses, dubbed 'environmental theories', suggests that syntax was selected for because it helped us to hunt game, or gather foodstuffs, or make better tools. But there are plenty of animals that hunt very well without having to talk about it. As for tool making, it is possible that there is a causal relationship between linguistic competence and manual dexterity. While tool development did, albeit very slowly, improve during the last two million years in which early hominids presumably developed a universal grammar, there was a sudden explosion of innovative tool making about 50,000 years ago. Corballis suggests that it was the emergence of a vocal apparatus (the lips, larynx, and tongue) physically capable of supporting speech independently of the rest of the body that freed the hands to make better tools. His is an interesting conjecture. But I think more likely than these general intelligence or environmental theories is a social explanation of linguistic evolution.

The anthropologist Robin Dunbar has pointed out that brain size in various primates correlates quite nicely with the average size of the social group, which, in turn, directly correlates with the amount of time individuals spend grooming one another. Humans have the largest brains per body weight, live amidst relatively large social groups and spend much of their time socializing. Even with an excellent memory, it is difficult to keep track of 150 people and constantly attend to their ever-changing needs and demands without the aid of some sort of language, whether gestural, spoken, or written. Dunbar believes that the demands of social life may have been the selection pressure driving the evolution of the language instinct.

I believe that grammar genes and linguistic brain circuits may indeed have evolved in response to the selective pressure of social intercourse. Language was selected for by the reproductive and/or survival advantage it conferred on those individuals who had it. The advantage is clear: the possession of universal grammar allows one to articulate thoughts, plans, warnings, and dreams to one's peers, relatives, friends, and rivals, allowing more effective and efficient allocation of know-how and resources. It is also a fabulous instrument of courtship; a fitness indicator par excellence that one can use to dazzle a future mate. Charming men use their wit to win wives. Charmed women find witty men irresistible. There is no reason to believe that our ancestors were any different.

Much of what we use language for has to do with comprehending and describing the relationships between different objects and agents, whether physical, biological, or psychological. Some of these relationships can become very complex. Imagine trying to formulate the phrase, 'this is the cow with the crumpled horn that tossed the dog that worried the cat that killed the rat that ate the malt that lay in the house that Jack built' without words. Words and their arrangement into grammatical phrases allow us to capture and convey the ins in outs of complex situations with surprising ease. This is made possible by recursive logic, the mental act of taking a nugget of information and embedding it into a larger nugget of information, which, in turn, can be embedded in an even larger nugget of information, and so on. Technically, there is no limit to the extent of recursion we can imagine and produce linguistically other than rules against awkward grammar, the limits of short-term memory, and the attention span of the listener.

Recursive logic is a central component of the language instinct. All languages from Gaelic to Greek, Farsi to Finn, ancient Sanskrit to Modern American Sign use it in one form or another. In fact, the ability to think recursively may have been the first step in the development of syntax. Recursive logic is also, as we have seen, a key component of Theory of Mind. TOM statements utilize the same recursive structures we find in embedded syntax. The difference is that TOM involves the additional element of mental states.

Are We Unique?
Folk physics, intuitive biology, Theory of Mind, recursive logic. How much of this is inherently human? Let's go down the checklist and see how other creatures measure up. It is clear that creatures as humble as fruit flies come equipped with high quality motion detection and object recognition software. Much more so than with humans, the code is pretty much written into their

hard drives, leaving relatively little room for learning. When it comes to face detection, all mammals and probably most birds are as good as humans, at least when it comes to detecting their own kind. Memory, both semantic and episodic, is also well developed in mammals, although the autobiographical component is probably considerably impoverished relative to ours considering the lack of self-consciousness in nonhuman species.

Things get more interesting when we get to agency detection. Recall that the ADD incorporates several different skill sets including eye direction/biological motion detection and emotional perception. These are all well developed in many mammals. Certainly, creatures like rats and monkeys depend on these signals for their very survival. It seems reasonable to assume that many animals, or at least mammals, do have a rudimentary form of innate psychology. But they can understand only what they perceive. Animals can treat and respond to other creatures 'as if' they were agents, but they have no concept of other minds because they can't even conceptualize their own mind.

The evolutionary psychologists Daniel Povinelli and Jennifer Vonk have done extensive research on the cognitive capacities of our closest living relatives, the chimpanzees. Their results are revealing. In the realm of intuitive physics, the chimps flunk. They do a pretty good job of associating one event with another, such as the shaking of a tree and the falling of fruit. They use this to predict the consequences of actions (either others' or their own). But they don't understand the concepts of inertia, or force at a distance, or object permanence, or the conservation of number, all of which a human infant grasps intuitively. Povinelli compared chimps and preschool children on a task in which they were to stack up some blocks. In one experiment, one of the blocks was visibly defective so that it tended to fall over. Both the children and the chimps inspected the faulty block. In the second experiment, one of the blocks was defective in another way: it was weighted to one side, but looked just like the others. Most of the children examined the sham block, but none of the chimps did. For chimpanzees – and some humans – it really is 'out of sight, out of mind'. The same seems to hold for intuitive biology. The human belief in essentialism does not apply to nonhuman creatures. To us, a wolf in sheep's clothing is still a wolf, but to a lamb, it's probably just another sheep (although this experiment would be difficult to do in practice). Appearance is everything; other animals cannot conceive of an underlying reality beneath their perceptions.

Finally, we reach the rarified realm of Theory of Mind. This is a contentious area, but there is as yet not enough evidence to suggest that the chimpanzee or any other nonhuman animal is capable of understanding false belief. In fact, there is no evidence to suggest that they are capable of recursive thought.

Even if animals had an ADD, without recursive logic, they cannot invent mathematics, language, or TOM. Human beings are unique in the animal kingdom in several ways. First, our minds have a natural ability to represent information in a Russian doll-like format, which in turn has given rise both to our language instinct and a TOMM. Second, we can conceptualize things that are not immediately accessible to our perceptual apparatus, thus enabling us to take extended virtual journeys stretching across expanses of space and time.

Genes and Development

Now it's time to get real. What exactly are the physical and biochemical correlates of psychological phenomena? What are the roots of thought? Fortunately, molecular geneticists and developmental biologists have traced those roots quite deep. Here is a quick rundown of eight important things to remember when looking at the mind from the top down.

First, all psychology and behavior can be reduced to manifestations of metabolic and computational activity (energetics and informatics) within the nervous system. **Second**, the nervous system develops from a brainless fertilized egg through complex interactions of genes and the environment in which the embryo eventually becomes an adult. **Third**, every neuron in every brain of all organisms contains a complete set of genetic information for building the entire organism. **Fourth**, although almost every cell in the body has the complete genome (made of nucleotide sequences strung out on chromosomes) on its hard drive, only some of this information is expressed during its lifetime; the specific pattern of gene expression determines not just what the cell does, but what the cell is.

Fifth, the when and where of gene expression is tightly controlled by complex networks of regulatory genes, called transcription factors, whose expression is regulated by still other transcription factors higher up on the hierarchy. **Sixth**, genetic software is expressed first as messenger RNA, and then as protein, the hardware that makes up the visible architecture of cells, brains, and bodies. **Seventh**, cells, brains, and bodies coalesce largely through the expression of hardwired genetic instructions, but there is plenty of wiggle room as epigenetics (non-genetic information contained within the chromatin), physiology, environment, and education play important roles in fine-tuning. **Eighth**, your genetic code is a living record of your ancestors' struggles to survive and reproduce. Every one of you who is alive is a success story: a living monument commemorating not just your own success, but the successes of all your forebears who mustered the strength and skill to pass on each and every one of the 20,000+ genes that you now carry in almost every cell of your body. All of those genes were selected in the course of evolution to build bodies and brains that enabled your ancestors to outcompete less successful rivals.

With these eight points in mind, let's start from the ground and work our way up. Our first stop is the long arm of the seventh human chromosome (7q). It is here that a gene called the *forkhead box P2* (FOXP2) is located. The story starts with a curious disorder of language processing first described in an English family, the KE's. Affected members of this family had normal education and intelligence, but they had difficulty speaking and writing with proper grammar, and they failed to comprehend spoken and written language above a rudimentary level. This disorder, dubbed 'specific language impairment' (SLI) was found to be inherited in an autosomal dominant pattern. In 1997, a team of geneticists from Oxford University used a technique called *linkage analysis* to localize the putative SLI gene to a small region of chromosome 7q. When FOXP2 itself was subsequently isolated, cloned, and sequenced a few years later, it was widely heralded as the discovery of the 'language gene'.

FOXP2 is a member of a large family of proteins called *transcription factors*. These proteins are designed to latch on to the regulatory regions of other genes (they have a DNA binding region on their business end specifically for this purpose), thereby increasing or decreasing the expression of the target gene's messenger RNA and protein product. Transcription factors are very common in human and other genomes, comprising upwards of ten percent of all genes. This would make sense given their importance as masters of transcription regulation. In the case of the KE family, the FOXP2 gene was found to have a mutation of just one nucleotide out of several thousand, but it was enough to render the entire protein defective. Children born with just one copy of the mutated FOXP2 gene suffer abnormal brain development, especially involving the speech and language centers on the left parietal lobe (Broca's area), which can be picked up on MRI scans.

SLI is an experiment of nature that offers science a terrific window into the molecular basis of language comprehension. Biologists have made mouse models of SLI by using an ingenious technique called *gene knockouts*. In short, here is how to make a knockout mouse (Figure 12). First, we start with a cloned copy of the mouse gene of interest, in this case, FOXP2. Mice and men share much DNA homology. Using standard recombinant DNA technology, we insert a gene that confers resistance to certain antibiotics into the middle of the FOXP2 gene. This has the dual effect of inactivating or 'knocking out' the gene of interest, and also allowing only those cells that happen to take up this synthetically created piece of DNA to survive antibiotic treatment. Second, this recombinant construct is then inserted into mice embryonic stem (ES) cells cultured from dark colored mice. Rarely, this construct will integrate into its correct or *homologous* site on the mouse cell's DNA. This is called a *targeted insertion*.

Those mouse ES cells with the targeted knockout insertion can then be selected using the antibiotic. Third, these cells are then inserted into otherwise healthy four-day-old light colored mouse embryos, called *blastocysts*, which are hollow balls of cells. The blastocysts are then reimplanted into a surrogate mother. The resulting mice pups will have a mixture of cells descended from the dark colored knockout ES cells, and cells of the light colored embryo into which the ES cells were inserted. It will have light and dark stripes of fur since the animal is a *mosaic* of cells from two different colored strains. Some, but not all, of these mosaics will have the knockout gene in their germline cells and can be used to produce offspring with one copy of the gene knocked out. Finally, to produce homozygous knockout mice mutant for FOXP2, we cross two mice with germline knockout mutations to each other.

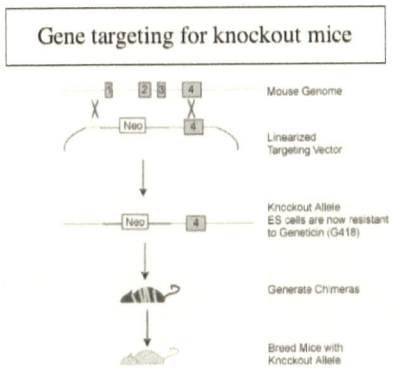

Figure 12

Once the FOXP2 knockouts have been generated, we can study the animals for behavioral, anatomical, and biochemical abnormalities. If these creatures display defective socialization or communication, it would suggest that we have created an animal model for SLI. The next step would be to localize the function of the protein temporally and spatially in the developing mouse. Scientists have perfected ingenious techniques to do this. They are called *conditional knockouts* and figure 13 shows how this is done. We start by crossing two different strains of genetically engineered mice. The first has a form of the gene of interest that can be deleted when treated with a specific enzyme called *cre recombinase*. The second is a *transgenic mouse* with a tissue specific promoter spliced to a gene for cre. Thus the hybrid knockout mice will have a defective copy of the gene only in those tissues *where* the promoter is active, such as the hippocampus, or basal ganglia, or amygdala, but not in the heart, or skin, or eye. Second, scientists can regulate *when* the gene is to be shut down during development by injecting a drug which activates the cre enzyme that deletes the gene. By shutting down the gene at different periods of development, we can see what behavioral and physiological abnormalities result in these conditional knockouts.

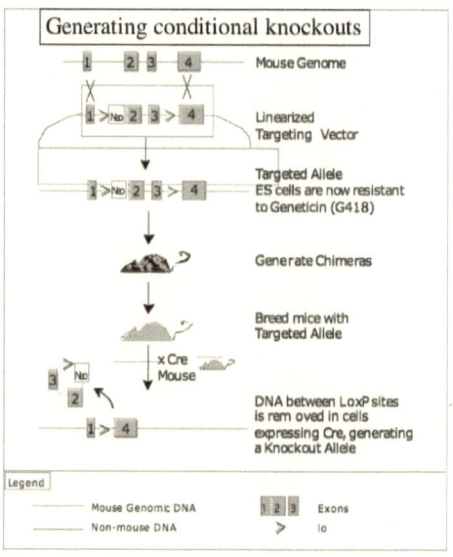

Figure 13

Finally, we can use knockout mice to find downstream effects of the initial mutation. Recall that dysfunctional transcription factors result in other genes being abnormally turned off or on. We can isolate total mRNA from these knockout animals, label it with a fluorescent tag, and pour the labeled mRNA over DNA microarrays or *gene chips* (now commercially available from Affymetrix) embedded with thousands of single stranded DNA copies of normal genes arranged in a two-dimensional array (Figure 14). If a specific mRNA is present in the tissue extract, it binds to its corresponding DNA on the wafer and lights it up. If not, the spot stays dark. A computer scans the chip and prints out the presence and intensity of each gene expression signal. Cutting edge technologies such as gene chips allow us to tell where, when, and how much of thousands of genes are expressed in development.

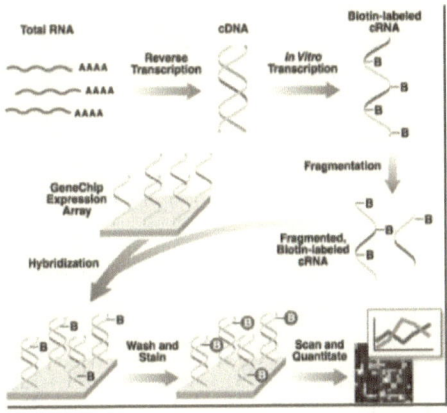

Figure 14: Gene chips

Heterozygous FOXP2 knockouts do indeed demonstrate decreased vocalization and impaired socialization when compared with other mice. Homozygous double knockouts suffer severe brain damage and die within twenty-one days of respiratory failure. This is not surprising as the FOXP2 gene is expressed in the lung as well as the brain. It is fair to conclude that human embryos with homozygous mutations are probably aborted early in pregnancy.

A final point about FOXP2 is its remarkable conservation throughout the course of evolution. The mouse version of the protein differs from our own by just three amino acids. The chimpanzee FOXP2 has just two different amino acids. But perhaps the most fascinating discovery was made by the evolutionary anthropologist Svante Pääbo at the University of Leipzig. In the course of his remarkable efforts to reconstruct the genome of the Neanderthal man, he found that these early humans' FOXP2 is identical to our own. Does this mean that Neanderthals could speak? We don't know for sure. While the gene does appear to be necessary for language, it is unclear if it is also sufficient. Probably not, given the complexity of the language instinct. What is clear is that despite our close genetic proximity to other mammals, and especially to the apes, small differences mean a lot. Think about it. Humans have twenty-three chromosomes with about 20,000 genes spanning some three billion base pairs of DNA. The fruit fly has 17,000 genes. The nematode worm has 14,000 genes. The lowly onion you buy in the supermarket has five billion base pairs in its genome. But most of us are smarter than flies, worms, and onions. Much of the difference can be explained by slight variations at the level of transcription factors like FOXP2. At the end of the day, the measure of our brain capacity lies not the sheer amount of DNA nor the number of genes we have, nor even the size of our brains, but in how those genes are regulated, the complexity of our genetic and neural networks, and our propensity to learn. Genes are very important, but we are more than our genes.

SLI and autism are separate disorders, but the co-occurrence of the two in affected families is considerable. Autism has been found to have a prevalence of 3% in siblings of SLI individuals, compared to 0.5% in the general population. Conversely, language disorders of various types are quite prevalent in families of autistic individuals. Autism itself is in many ways a disorder of communication. A quarter of first-degree relatives of autistic children experience speech delay or reading problems as compared to about 5% to 10% in the general population. But unlike SLI, autism also involves a defective TOMM. This brings us to the genetic basis of TOM.

Autism is a genetic disorder. It is not caused by vaccines, or bad parenting, or a bump on the head; it is caused by mutated genes. Like SLI, autism tends to cluster within families. But unlike more straightforward genetic diseases like cystic fibrosis or Huntington's disease, autism is a complex disorder involving dozens of defective genes scattered randomly throughout the genome. Progress has been tough; genome-wide screens have failed to turn out more than a few possible leads. It appears that autism is not caused by a few common genetic mutants, but by many very uncommon ones. Fortunately, one of them has been found.

There is a rare genetic disorder on the autism spectrum called *Rett syndrome*. Rett differs from common autism in that it affects primarily girls and has a prevalence of one in ten thousand. Common autism affects as many as one in two hundred and has a male/female ratio of four to one (the related *Asperger syndrome* is ten times more common in boys). Kids with Retts have relatively normal cognitive development for the first six months of life, but then start to suffer from seizures, growth retardation, motor problems, and severe autistic symptoms. Unlike typical autism, Rett is caused by a single defective gene. This gene is located on the long arm of the X chromosome (Xq28) and codes for a protein called *methyl CpG binding protein 2* or simply, *MeCP2*. And you guessed it, it's a transcription factor. The protein is unique among transcription factors in that its mechanism of action is to bind to methylated sites on cytosine residues adjacent to guanine (CpG sites). Many genes have clusters of these sites in so-called *CpG islands*, which make convenient targets for MeCP2. Once bound, the gene is physically tied up by large protein spools called *histones* and thereby silenced. But MeCP2 can also turn on other genes by a different mechanism. MeCP2 is expressed at a high level in nerve cells, and is thought to play a major role in synaptic plasticity.

Biologists have recently constructed MeCP2 knockout mice. These 'Rett mice' developed into adults that displayed classic traits of autism such as twirling around endlessly and avoiding social contact with other mice. In a further twist, Professor Rudolph Jaenish of MIT extended the original experiment by taking these autistic adult rodents and then knocking the MeCP2 gene *back in*. Remarkably, these modified Rett mice seemed to be 'cured' of their autism. Although this technique, which requires the manipulation of embryos, is not directly applicable to humans on technical (and moral) grounds, it does imply that the miswiring of the autistic brain may not have to be a permanent condition.

The above experiments suggest that genes like MeCP2 may be necessary (but not sufficient) for a dedicated Theory of Mind module. By turning on and off the right genes at the right times in the right places in the developing brain, transcription factors allow proper synaptogenesis, synaptic plasticity, and the pruning of unwanted connections. A well-connected, specialized brain is essential for any cognitive process as complex as language and TOM. It is not clear when TOM evolved, but we have a pretty good idea as to where it may reside. Neuroimaging studies done on experimental subjects performing TOM tests suggest that the critical locus is in the *right prefrontal cortex*. This roughly corresponds to the language center in Broca's area, which is located in the *left prefrontal cortex*. This invites the intriguing possibility that both TOM and syntax evolved simultaneously in opposite but corresponding parts of the brain, as our early hominid ancestors learned to capitalize on some serendipitous genetic mutations that enabled recursive, embedded thoughts to occur in their brains.

This is an exciting time as the two major branches of modern biology, gene science and brain science, are now finally joining forces to discover and investigate many genes like FOXP2 and MeCP2 that are directly involved in the wiring up of the developing brain. If we really want to find out how and where cognitive modules like face detectors, agency detection devices, recursive logic, language instincts, Theory of Mind detectors, and anything else necessary for magical and spiritual thinking do their special jobs, we will need to see how the relevant neurons are hooked up, and 'who' directs the construction of all the wires and connections. Ultimately, these are questions that only well-trained and disciplined molecular geneticists and neurobiologists can answer with rigorous experiments, not over-zealous cognitive psychologists and armchair anthropologists with wild speculations.

Religious Universals

There are at least seven characteristic themes that are common to all religions. Their universality suggests that they were deeply embedded in the evolutionary foundations of the first proto-religions. These are:

- Belief that the body is separate from the mind
- Belief that life has a purpose
- Belief in a supernatural creator who listens to and cares for the believer
- Rules to live by
- Taboos
- Rituals
- Displays of sacrifice and commitment

I believe that if we can create a coherent account for the origins of these seven components, we can make a case for the evolutionary basis of religion.

First up is the old concept of mind/body dualism, an illusion I tried to demolish in the first chapter. Unfortunately it's alive and well in the guise of religion. Religious people everywhere (and perhaps some non-religious ones, too) are convinced that their minds, thoughts, memories, or some evanescent essence thereof will somehow survive the physical destruction of their bodies and live on as immaterial spirits. Different religions vary as to the precise nature and behavior of these spirits. Christians maintain that all people have souls that end up in heaven, hell, or a temporary halfway house called purgatory after their death. They are rather vague on the precise location of these places, but it was commonly believed until quite recently that heaven was somewhere in the upper atmosphere and hell lurked deep under the earth's crust. The Vatican has, however, officially rescinded the existence of purgatory.

Buddhists also believe in souls, but they give them the luxury of mobility based on merit. A spirit needs a physical vehicle, and can be reborn as another human, animal, or even a vegetable or rock, depending on one's behavior in the previous life. Practitioners of Afro-Caribbean voodoo cults such as *Santería* take this further and maintain that bodies and souls can be separated or re-combined even before death, resulting in living bodies without souls (zombies), souls without bodies (ghosts), or bodies possessed by alien souls. People of many faiths claim the ability to communicate and interact with the spiritual world while in trance-like states of altered consciousness. In fact, traversing this divide through prayer, meditation, hypnosis, or the ingestion of mind-altering chemicals is the cherished cornerstone of religious practice.

All religious systems from primitive tribal cults of remote highland New Guinea to the great monotheistic faiths of the Near East offer their members answers to those awesome questions about meaning and purpose. Invariably, the goal of life is the renunciation of the physical world, both its pleasures and pains, in preparation for something immeasurably greater to follow. Jews, Christians, and Muslims alike believe that those who adhere to the teachings of their holy books will find salvation and unity with their creator. According to the Hindu *Upanishads*, life's purpose is to liberate one's soul from the endless and vicious cycle of *karma* (causality), thereby achieving *moksha* (unity) with *Brahman* (the incarnation of cosmic reality). Similarly, the Theravada Buddhists maintain that if one is able to focus, through education and meditation, on transcending the inevitable sufferings of everyday life, then one can attain *Nirvana* (the state of mental perfection). The commonality among all these theological systems is that the meaning of life is tied to finding our place within the greater cosmos, and conversely, the purpose of the universe is to find its way into our minds.

This brings us to the concept of God(s). All cultures ever studied have a creation mythology purporting to explain the origins of life, the universe, and mankind. Seven centuries before Christ, the Greek poet Hesiod penned the Theogony, in which he writes of Chaos giving birth to Gaea (the earth), Tartarus (the underworld), Eros (desire), Nyx (the darkness of night), and Erebus (the darkness of the underworld). From them were conceived all the other gods of Greek mythology. Hesiod almost certainly adopted these stories from an oral tradition dating back several centuries before that. The very first recorded creation myth comes to us from the ancient Sumerians of Mesopotamia. The Eridu Genesis cuneiform tablet, which dates back some eighteen centuries before the Christian era, tells the story of Enki, the god of the waters, who unleashed a terrible flood that wiped out all humans except the hero, Zi-ud-sura, and his wife. The couple subsequently repopulated the world with their seed and those of the animals they saved on a giant boat they were instructed to build. This fable was later adopted by the Jewish scribes who penned the story of Noah in the Old Testament. There are scores of narratives like this in all cultures throughout the world. They all attempt to link the creation of an unconscious, impersonal physical universe to the intentions of conscious, purposeful supernatural beings. These gods are rather humanlike in their motivations, emotions, and sometimes also their physical forms, and they seem to care about and interact with the ordinary people who believe in them.

All religions are a source of ethics as well as metaphysics. As such, they come with elaborate sets of rules and regulations about what can and cannot be done, along with equally elaborate rewards and punishments for obeying or transgressing them. Despite regional variations, they're all pretty much the same. Points are given for fairness and reciprocation, refraining from excessive violence and thuggery, respect for authority (parents, elders, chiefs), faithfulness to husbands (perhaps less so for wives), and avoidance of contaminated food and drink. Points are deducted for selfishness, violation of others' property (including wives), and, especially, disrespecting the gods.

These rules and taboos were passed down for generations through sermons and lectures from parents, teachers, shamans, and priests, and, after the invention of papyrus, paper, and printing press, through the circulation of holy texts. But the most effective means of reinforcement is through ritual. And there is no shortage of that in the religions of the world. Devout Moslems prostrate themselves five times a day facing the general direction of Mecca; Catholics repeat the Hail Mary twenty five times while fiddling with their rosaries; Jews lose themselves in rhythmic head-bobbing at the Western Wall; Southern Baptists burst into wild song and dance each Sunday. Despite all their obsessive-compulsive energy expenditure, most rituals are relatively benign. Not so with ritual sacrifice.

Modern monotheistic faiths may have toned down some of their more egregiously spectacular displays of sacrifice, but don't be fooled. Hundreds of millions of believers devote hours or entire afternoons of potential leisure or self-enrichment time each week sitting on hard benches or concrete floors listening to lies about salvation and the afterlife. They mindlessly discard much of their hard earned money into church coffers. They sacrifice food, clothing, and shelter at fundraisers. But things used to be much worse. All tribal religions, at least before the great age of European imperialism, practiced human sacrifice. The Aztecs and Maya of Mexico were notorious for the scale and brutality of their sacrificial ceremonies. The entire Judeo-Christian narrative is founded on Abraham's willingness to sacrifice his son Isaac on the Rock of Jerusalem (later the site of the First and Second Jewish Temples, and now the site of the Al-Aksa Mosque). Christianity itself is centered on God's sacrifice of his son on the Cross. The Dani people of New Guinea still chop off parts of their fingers to satisfy the souls of departed loved ones. Hindus run a brisk business of animal sacrifice at their temple at Varanasi. Sacrifice is simply part and parcel of religious life.

Spandrel Theory: Mixing the Modules

In the beginning, God created the earth and every living creature and one was man. Mud as man alone could speak. God leaned close as mud as man sat up, and spoke. 'What is the purpose of this?' he asked politely.

'Everything must have a purpose?' asked God.

'Certainly', said man.

'Than I leave it to you to think of one for all this', said God.

And He went away.

The Book of Bokonon

from <u>Cat's Cradle</u> by Kurt Vonnegut

With his masterpiece, <u>Meditations on the First Philosophy</u>, Rene Descartes brought mind/body dualism to the forefront of Western Philosophy. What he didn't know was that his ancestors had already been practicing it for a hundred thousand years or more. In fact, all non-autistic children become dualists by the time they reach four years of age. As I explained earlier, infants start to develop an innate understanding of the physical world before their first birthday. Meanwhile, they undergo a parallel development of intuitive psychology that culminates in a full-fledged Theory of Mind by the time they reach kindergarten. According to cognitive psychologist Paul Bloom of Yale, author of <u>Descartes' Baby</u>, these two worldviews are in conflict. On the one hand, one can accept the fact that material objects have mass, kinetic energy, form, texture, compressibility, and so forth. On the other hand, one can also believe that they feel pain, pleasure, hunger, and fear, have hopes and dreams, and remember their past experiences. But how come some things fall into only the first category, while others also belong to the second? The child's mind comes to the conclusion that there must be two different kinds of objects. Adults should know better, but most of us never totally outgrow this false belief. For someone naïve to the concepts of molecular genetics and cortico-thalamic re-entry loops (which pretty much includes the vast majority of people throughout the vast majority of human history), dualism is the natural way out. Folk physics + folk psychology = dualism.

Now add the agency detection device. Recall that the ADD is a cognitive module that evolved in our remote ancestors as a result of selective pressure to avoid being eaten by stealthy predators. It works by taking advantage of the intentional stance (treating something as an agent with beliefs, desires, and choices). A simple example is the assumption that the rustling of leaves is a tiger lying in wait, rather than, well, the rustling of leaves.

The ADD was so useful that for most of us, it's become overactive. Psychologist Justin Barrett of Cambridge University has coined the term hyperactive agency detection device (HADD) to refer to the natural tendency to attribute beliefs, desires, and intentions onto mindless objects. Whenever we curse our bum knee, or try to coax our dubious car engine back to life, the HADD is busy at work. The combination of the HADD and dualistic thinking inevitably leads to the belief in spirits, souls, and ghosts. HADD + dualism = belief in spirits. When applied to the death of a loved one, the results are particularly dramatic. Dan Dennett goes into some detail in his book, <u>Breaking the Spell: Religion as a Natural Phenomenon</u>.

> 'When somebody we love or even just know well dies, we suddenly are confronted with a major task of cognitive updating: revising all our habits of thought to fit a world with one less familiar intentional system in it. "I wonder if she'd like…," "Does she know I'm…," "Oh, look, this is something she always wanted…" A considerable portion of the pain and confusion we suffer when confronting a death is caused by the frequent, even obsessive, reminders that our intentional stance habits throw up at us like annoying pop-up ads but much, much worse.
>
> 'But there is a problem: a corpse is a potent source of disease, and we have evolved a strong compensatory innate disgust mechanism to make us keep our distance. Pulled by longing and pushed back by disgust, we are in turmoil when we confront the corpse of a loved one. Small wonder that this crisis should play so central a role in the birth of religions everywhere.'

We have explained the belief in spirits, the afterlife, and funeral ceremonies in terms of overactive cognitive processes like agency detectors, Theory of Mind modules, and disgust reactions. These processes are encoded in dedicated brain circuits that are constructed by specific genes that evolved in our ancestors in response to selective pressures to survive and mate in genuinely dangerous social and physical environments. But they did not evolve for the particular purpose of allowing us to believe in imaginary things like ghosts, reincarnation, or heaven. These functions came along as evolutionary by-products or 'spandrels'. This wonderful term comes to us from architecture and art history. The spandrel is the empty space between the top of an arch and its rectangular enclosure, commonly seen on bridges and churches. The spandrel serves no structural or functional purpose for the building itself, but is routinely used for decorative sculptures (friezes), which, of course, can have a separate function on their own.

Like the belief in souls, the concept of God and the meaning of life are spandrels spun off the evolution of the human mind. It starts with teleological thinking: the notion that things and events in nature have purpose. The psychologist Deborah Kelemen has confirmed something that all parents and teachers already know: children describe the world teleologically. When she asked a typical four year-old why it rains, the child replied, "so that plants can have water to grow". Likewise, other children said that clouds are for raining, mountains are for climbing, lions are for zoos, and, my favorite, pointy rocks are for animals to scratch their backs on. Children employ teleological explanations much more than adults do. Kelemen and her colleagues then tested nursing home residents suffering from Alzheimer's disease. They, too, were more teleologically-minded than normal adults. Two conclusions can be drawn from these studies. First, there is an innate teleological module that normally comes on-line by age four and governs how children think the world works. Second, teleological thought is largely overridden by acquired background knowledge in adults, but those with dementia sometimes fall back on it. It may be that teleological thinking is the default setting of the human mind in the absence of a better explanation.

The teleological module, like the agency detection device, was selected in the course of human evolution because it helped our ancestors predict the future. It is often quite helpful from a motivational standpoint to believe that some things (water holes, sharp sticks) are there for a reason (drinking, self-defense). The ability to think teleologically was so useful, in fact, that people, especially young children, the demented, and the uneducated, often overuse it. Ironically, one consequence of a hyperactive teleology module is the failure to grasp the relatively straightforward concept of evolution by natural selection. According to the teleological argument, all living things were created for a reason, hence the need for an intelligent designer. The fact that a blind process like Darwinism can result in the baroque complexity of life on earth seems counterintuitive not just to children, who are natural born creationists, but also to the billions of adults worldwide who are ignorant of science. Another consequence of teleological hyperactivity is the idea that all things in the cosmos, including oneself, have a reason for being. The teleological mind demands an existential explanation. In its absence, one will simply have to be created.

I think that the widespread illusion that one's life has meaning and purpose is a spandrel effect of hyperactive teleological thinking (probably localized to the prefrontal cortex) combined with an activated limbic system (centered on the temporal cortex and amygdala). Both neural centers are necessary. The prefrontal circuits allow one to conceptualize the connection between cause and effect, the universe and its origins, life and its purpose. The limbic circuits imbue those connections with believability.

What about God? That too can be explained by the mixing of cognitive modules. If we combine creationism, a product of teleological hyperactivity, with spirits, which come from a HADD, we invariably end up with the notion of a creating spirit. We're almost there. But in most religions, God is more than just an omniscient, all-powerful creator; He/She/It is also someone who (sometimes) cares for you and listens to your prayers. In other words, He possesses both a mind of His own, as well as a theory of your mind. This fits quite nicely with the TOMM. To summarize, hyperactive teleology = creationism; HADD = spirits; creationism + spirits + TOMM = personal God.

Language's Infinite Leash

Common wisdom has it that language constrains the mind. For example, 'Words can't begin to describe how I feel', 'words get in the way', 'words are never enough', and so on. At one point in the history of linguistics, there was a lively debate as to whether it was even possible to have thoughts without language [it is]. Language does, however, put some limits on the kind of thoughts that can readily be expressed. As I noted earlier, every language is patterned according to the rules of innate syntax. Universal grammar is not a direct-matching mechanism that allows every quantum of thought to be paired with a corresponding symbolic gesture, but rather involves a genetically based cognitive trick called recursive logic. Like TOM, language is good for packaging coherent thought streams in embedded form.

More importantly, language liberates thought. It allows an infinite number of distinct sentences, each of which carries a distinct meaning. Moreover, words and phrases streamline otherwise unruly thoughts into neat packages which can be easily recalled, rehearsed, and transmitted to other minds. Finally, when harnessed to the TOMM and the creativity generator in the prefrontal cortex, language can express the full range of the human imagination. To paraphrase the sociobiologist, E.O. Wilson, if our genes hold culture on a leash, language then stretches that leash to infinity.

Examples of language's long leash abound in religious catchphrases the world over. Here are just a few from the English version of the Judeo-Christian lexicon: 'Thank God', 'What the hell', 'God damn it', 'God bless you', 'may the Lord have mercy on your soul', and so on. There are thousands of others in every language and from every faith. But while diverse, these phrases are still limited to several recurring key themes, namely, God, souls, rules, and rituals. This reflects the underlying mental landscape that originally gave rise to the spoken and later written word. No matter how flexible the language, we cannot express what we cannot conceive. While one could speak of mind-reading time-traveling intergalactic dildos, giant one-eyed flying spaghetti monsters, or better yet, colorless green ideas that sleep furiously, we don't do that because those are not the things that our minds have been selected to think about. Our mental organs prefer more conservative and less imaginative fairy tales like the disembodied voice of an old man commanding people to sacrifice their first-born, winged steeds flying deftly across the Arabian night, and prophets transforming water into wine. Even the most hardened atheists probably delighted in childhood bedtime stories of talking toads, sleeping beauties, mischievous leprechauns, and flying reindeer. God could be something very bizarre like a nine-dimensional string vibrating at the frequency of Planck space-time, but He is usually depicted as quite human-like because even our imagination needs something to hang its hat on.

To take a page from the dualist handbook, our physical bodies inhabit a world of wind, water, and fire but our minds inhabit a psychological realm that is no less real. And just as our physical bodies are naturally selected by the contingencies of the real world in which we live, our minds and brains are naturally selected by the contingencies of the virtual worlds in which we think. The evolutionary biologist Richard Dawkins expresses this notion beautifully in his book, Unweaving the Rainbow:

> 'We move through a virtual world of our own brains' making. Our constructed models of rocks and of trees are a part of the environment in which we animals live, no less than the real rocks and trees that they represent. And, intriguingly, our virtual worlds must also be seen as part of the environment in which our genes are naturally selected… In the case of highly social animals like ourselves and our ancestors, our virtual worlds are, at least in part, group constructions. Especially since the invention of language and the rise of artifact and technology, our genes have had to survive in complex and changing worlds for which the most economical description we can find is shared virtual reality. It is a startling thought that, just as genes can be said to survive in deserts or forests, and just as they can be said to survive in the company of other genes in the gene pool, genes can also be said to survive in the virtual, even poetic worlds created by brains.'

All complex adaptations, whether biological, neurological, or cultural are the products of Darwinian selection. The fundamental laws of physics and chemistry are profoundly powerful in helping us to understand things like the formation of galaxies and the behavior of subatomic particles, but are too general to explain the kinds of complexity found in biology, psychology, and human culture. These are emergent historical phenomena emanating from Darwinian selection.

Natural selection is one kind of Darwinian process, but not the only possible kind. Biological evolution depends on the replication of DNA. Other kinds of selection may involve other very different replicators. This is the concept of *universal Darwinism*. The basic principles of variation, heredity, and selection are the same, but the nature of the replicator is different. As I mentioned in the first chapter, the brain itself may use a kind of replication of synaptic patterns to generate coherent mental states. Extraterrestrial life, if it exists, is likely to involve Darwinian selection involving a non-DNA based replication system. If artificially intelligent machines can one day be made to self-replicate, perhaps using a silicon-based code, they, too, would necessarily be subjected to Darwinian selection. Likewise, cultural evolution might undergo Darwinian selection, independent of the genes. I believe that the combination of a HADD, a hyperactive teleology module, TOM, and language results in a mental landscape ripe for infection by a second replicator.

Mental Viruses

At the end of his now classic book <u>The Selfish Gene</u>, Richard Dawkins introduced the term, *meme*, referring to a unit of cultural inheritance. Memes are packets of information: a line of poetry, a bit of political ideology or religious dogma, a recipe for shepherd's pie, the directions on how to copy a gesture, a tune, or a dance step, that are stored in the minds of individual people and then transferred to and replicated in others. Memes are selected for replication based on their usefulness or simply on their opportunistic ability. Quite a few animals are able to mimic gestures and behaviors. Recall those remarkable vervet monkeys. But only humans transmit and reproduce meaningful patterns of behavior readily and profusely using the media of spoken, written, and now electronic code. Language allows us to encode the instructions for doing or making something (the meme or *memotype*) into a unit of 'high fidelity, fecundity, and longevity' (the expressed meme *phenotype*). In this sense, memes are analogous to genes: they are the units of cultural heredity that undergo spontaneous variation, replication, and selection and are subject to competition and cooperation with other memes. Memes are a second replicator.

Dan Dennett believes that the human ability to propagate memes using language has opened up a whole new landscape of cultural design space: an arena for conceptual and behavioral patterns not bound by biological constraints. Here he critiques E.O. Wilson's gene centered view of culture:

> '...Wilson's leash is indefinitely long and elastic. Consider the huge space of *imaginable* cultural entities, practices, values. Is there any point in that Vast space that is utterly unreachable? Not that I can see. The constraints Wilson speaks of can be so co-opted, exploited, and blunted in a recursive cascade of

cultural products and meta-products that there may well be
traversable paths to every point in that space of imaginable
possibilities. I am suggesting, that is, that cultural possibility
is less constrained than genetic possibility. We can articulate
persuasive biological arguments to the effect that certain
imaginable species are unlikely in the extreme- flying
horses, unicorn, talking trees, carnivorous cows, spiders the
size of whales- but neither Wilson nor anybody else to my
knowledge has yet offered parallel grounds for believing
that there are similar obstacles to trajectories in imaginable
cultural design space. Many of these imaginable points in
design space would no doubt be genetic cul-de-sacs, in the
sense that any lineage of H. sapiens that ever occupied them
would eventually go extinct as a result, but this dire prospect
is no barrier to the evolution and adoption of such memes
in the swift time of cultural history. To combat Wilson's
metaphor with one of my own: the genes provide not a
leash but a launching pad, from which you can get almost
anywhere, by one devious route or another. It is precisely in
order to explain the patterns in cultural evolution that are
not strongly constrained by genetic forces that we need the
memetic approach.' [Dennett, "The evolution of culture",
the Charles Simonyi Lecture, Oxford University, Feb 17,
1999]

Consider the following. There is a single celled parasite called *Toxoplasma
gondii* (sounds like, but no relation to, the Mahatma) that infects most species
of mammals including up to *forty percent* of the human race. In the vast
majority of cases, the infections are relatively mild, causing some self-limited
flu-like symptoms or no symptoms at all. It is only dangerous to people with
weakened immune systems, such as those co-infected with HIV, patients
on chemotherapy, or infants born to infected mothers. But it has recently
come to light that otherwise asymptomatic people harboring the organism
may undergo subtle personality changes that may make them more likely to
engage in risk taking behavior such as reckless driving and promiscuous sex.
What's going on here?

Toxoplasma's preferred host is the cat (or other members of the feline
family). Only in the cat's gut can the microorganism reproduce sexually, after
which the resulting daughter cells or *oocysts* are excreted. When an animal
such as a rat eats food contaminated with toxoplasma-laden cat feces, the
oocysts hatch and enter the bloodstream, through which some of the parasites

eventually end up the brain. But the problem is that toxoplasma cannot have sex inside the rat. It 'wants' to get back into the cat. How this tiny brainless creature manages to accomplish this is yet another example of the remarkable elegance and ingenuity of natural selection.

It turns out that the parasite is attracted not just to the nervous system in general, but to one tiny part of the rat's brain: the amygdala. Once it migrates there, toxoplasma synthesizes and releases an enzyme called tyrosine hydroxylase, which, as I mentioned in the last chapter, is part of the pathway for the biosynthesis of dopamine. The resulting increase in dopamine concentration counteracts the natural tendency of the amygdala to produce fear. But what is truly remarkable is that in the case of the infected rats, it is *specifically the fear of cats* that is lost. The precise mechanism through which this linkage happens is unknown. The noted neuroendocrinologist and author Robert Sapolsky, who happens to be a Jewish atheist, has found that infected rats are actually attracted to the odor of cat urine, making them fearless enough to approach a hungry feline. In his words, "the cat's thinking, 'damn I'm good', the rat's thinking, 'what am I doing?', and toxoplasma is thinking, 'mission accomplished!'" These rats otherwise perform normally on tests of memory and cognition (maze tests) and exhibit the same nervous withdrawals to other threats. By evolving to commandeer the brains, minds, and behavior of the host, this parasite is able to reproduce and pass on the genes that allow it to do so to the next generation.

Human brains are also routinely infected by toxoplasma. But we haven't been around long enough to develop the same kind of relationship that cats or rats have with the parasite. We are accidental hosts. As such, infected humans aren't especially attracted to the odor of cat piss and don't approach wild lions without fear. But toxoplasma can alter our minds just as well. There is evidence that people with asymptomatic toxoplasma infections display impaired attention, slower reaction times, and more antisocial behavior. There is also evidence that infections are linked to higher rates of schizophrenia and bipolar disorder, which is not surprising considering the effect on dopamine concentrations. But none of these pathologies are beneficial for the parasite. Antisocial, psychotic, and life-threatening behavior doesn't get toxoplasma into cat guts. Human manifestations of toxoplasma infection are simply spandrels. Just as biological parasites like toxoplama can alter the minds of animals for the benefit of their genes, cultural parasites like religion can alter the minds of humans for the benefit of their memes.

Dennett makes an interesting analogy between the relationship of memes and their human hosts on the one hand, and parasites like toxoplasma and their biological hosts on the other. Some meme expressions, such as the practice of washing hands after using the bathroom, benefit both the host and the meme. These 'mutualistic memes' are somewhat analogous to the mutually beneficial relationship between toxoplasma and cats. Other meme expressions, such as humming a tune while waiting for the elevator or saying 'gesundheit!' when someone sneezes, have a neutral effect on the host. These are 'commensal' memes, analogous to toxoplasma's role in most asymptomatic human infections (although the recent evidence I mentioned above is beginning to question this view). Finally, some meme expressions are like toxoplasma's effect on infected rats: they are harmful to the host. These include celibacy, drug abuse, and warfare. These are 'parasitic' memes that benefit at the cost of the host's genes. It is easy to see why evolutionary psychologists would classify mutualistic and even commensal memes as cultural artifacts on genetic leashes. It is much harder for them to explain away parasitic memes using a 'gene's eye view'.

If a wildly successful but extremely pernicious parasitic meme, such as a policy of mutual assured nuclear destruction or the burning of carbon-based fuels leading to global warming, managed to infect and destroy the human race, then the meme itself would die out along with the genes simply because there would be no more human minds and bodies left to infect. But generally, like most biological parasites, parasitic memes are not quite as virulent for the host's genes. Genes and memes tend to co-evolve. Genes evolve to 'track' the evolution of memes so that their mutual host (the person who passes on the memes and the genes) stays alive and healthy enough to continue replicating the memes (through linguistic discourse) and the genes (through sexual intercourse). The problem now is that in this day of instant text messaging, Facebook, You Tube, Twitter, and the like, memes reproduce and evolve much faster (seconds, minutes, and days) than genes ever can (decades, centuries, and millennia). As a result, genes eventually lose track of the memes. To continue this metaphor, the leash that holds the memes grows longer and longer, until the memes simply break free.

Culture, language, and perhaps consciousness itself are vast collections of memes that sometimes cooperate and sometimes compete with one another for space in our brains and the opportunity to reproduce by commandeering our communicative organs. Like genes, which cooperate to produce organisms, memes can cooperate to produce cultures.

The Meme Theory of Religion

So what does all this talk of memes have to do with religion? Plenty, it turns out. The natural selection of genes for creating the architecture of a human brain that is best equipped to keep those genes alive also results in minds vulnerable to infection by certain memes. Once those memes have taken over the mind, they, in turn, become subject to selection creating the kinds of minds that are best equipped to keep those memes alive. When we deal with something as universal to human culture as religion, the question we need to ask is 'who benefits: genes or memes?' Dawkins and Dennett are decorated fellows of the Memetic School of religion. Steven Pinker, Pascal Boyer, and Scott Atran are somewhat less enthusiastic about memes. Their loyalty lies with the genetic spandrel camp. What they all have in common, however, is that none of them believe in the genetic advantage of religion. But in his book, The God Delusion, Dawkins makes the point that the spandrel theory and meme theory are not mutually exclusive:

> 'Organized religions are organized by people: by priests and bishops, rabbis, imams and ayatollahs. But...that doesn't mean they were conceived and designed by people. Even where religions have been exploited and manipulated to the benefit of powerful individuals, the strong possibility remains that the detailed form of each religion has been largely shaped by unconscious evolution. Not by genetic natural selection, which is too slow to account for the rapid evolution and divergence of religions. The role of genetic natural selection in the story is to provide the brain with its predilections and biases- the hardware platform and low-level system software which form the background to memetic selection. Given this background, memetic natural selection of some kind seems to me to offer a plausible account of the detailed evolution of particular religions. In the early stages of a religion's evolution, before it becomes organized, simple memes survive by virtue of their universal appeal to human psychology. This is where the meme theory of religion and the psychological by-product theory of religion overlap. The later stages, where a religion becomes organized, elaborate and arbitrarily different from other religions, are quite well handled by the theory of memeplexes – cartels of mutually compatible memes.'

We have discussed how genes prime brains capable of magical thoughts like the afterlife, divine creation, and cosmic meaning. But how about the other religious universals: rules, rituals, taboos, and sacrifice? I think meme theory is much better at explaining those. Take the case of the Hebrew Ten Commandments. Five of them are unquestionably beneficial for genetic survival: honor your parents, don't kill, don't steal, and don't bear false witness, on the grounds that following them protects civic order and breaking them usually results in retaliation and grievous physical punishment for the violator. Two of them are somewhat questionable: don't commit adultery and don't covet your neighbor's wife, but remember, these rules were written by men who lived in a time when women were basically private property, and offenders were punished accordingly. But the first three commandments confer absolutely no genetic benefit whatsoever: 'I am the Lord, your God, and you shall not worship any idols before me; don't take the name of God in vein; keep the Sabbath holy'. What does it matter that I worship Jesus Christ, or Vishnu, or Wotan, or Isis, or Aphrodite, or Santa Claus, or the Flying Spaghetti Monster, or last month's Playboy centerfold as long as I can continue to fuck my wife and make babies? Why do I have to keep Fridays or Saturdays or Sundays holy as long as I get enough rest to keep my mind and body fresh enough to pass on my genes? After all, it's much more relaxing to have a romantic cuddle in bed than to rush off to temple all the time and sacrifice my limited time and energy.

The logical explanation is that these rules (literally written in stone thousands of years ago) are memes that insured their own perpetuation. Think about it. What if the first three commandments said, 'you can worship anyone (or no one) as you please', 'you can use the word God (or any other word) as an exclamation whenever the urge strikes you', 'take a day of rest whenever you feel sick or tired'. Those would be more sensible and beneficial for our minds and our genes. But they would also be disastrous for the memes. If left unchecked, those revised commandments would spread like a bad virus throughout the population because people would prefer them to the original. The original memeplex that constituted the entire religious edifice would be undermined. In short, the religion would self-destruct.

A major reason why religions endure despite harboring doctrines that insult the intelligence and subjugate the minds and bodies of their adherents is that many of the memes, masquerading as rules and regulations, are also beneficial for the health of the genes. Examples include: 'thou shalt not kill', 'cleanliness is next to godliness', 'the road to heaven is paved with good intentions'. Memes that promote peace, hard work, social order, and public health are more likely to allow freeloading despotic memes that travel with them to survive.

Another reason for religion's resilience is that many of the rituals associated with it are actually enjoyable because they tap into the innate human propensity for rhythm expressed as dance, music, and chant. Just look at the remarkable kaleidoscope of rituals, festivals, services, and prayers inherent in every faith; they are full of rhythm and music. Orthodox Jews rocking at the Western Wall, Charismatic Christians dancing in the aisles, Roman Catholics gesticulating the Sign of the Cross and tripped out kids gyrating on the dance floor are all stimulating the same neural circuits. The reciprocating circuits in the basal ganglia are programmed to respond best to repetitive stimuli. Input, whether musical or visual, that resonates with the internal frequency of the motor circuit, gets amplified and makes us want to move. But re-entrant circuits are not limited to the motor system. They are found throughout the brain, including the amygdala/limbic system, and even the cortex, where they give rise to embodied cognition and consciousness itself. When an emotionally charged stimulus is captured by the limbic system and resonates at its frequency, that signal too will be amplified and linger in the mind. I believe this is the origin of the metaphors used to describe an emotionally powerful story as gripping, touching, or moving.

Related to this is religion's indelible stamp on things that appeal to our innate sense of beauty, which may itself be a spandrel of cognitive evolution. You don't have to believe in God to enjoy Dante's Inferno, or feel haunted by Grünewald's Isenheim Altarpiece, or be moved by Bach's Oratorio, or marvel at the grandeur of Saint Peter's Basilica. Religious or not, we find these things sublime because they are designed to push our pleasure buttons. Religions gain a major advantage by commandeering works of art as their own.

A final reason that religions survive is that many of their less savory war-like memes actually help to defend the rest of their meme cartel from competing belief systems. Millions have been slain by soldiers of faith inspired by rousing memes like 'By the sword of Allah, conquer', and 'I fight in the name of God and country'. The judicious use of beneficial memes, pleasurable memes, and aggressive memes in the guise of rules, rituals, and battle cries have allowed those religions that have survived the centuries to out-compete their rivals.

It is worth mentioning that just as religious universals such as the belief in the afterlife are by-products of genetic misfiring, certain cultural phenomena may be by-products of memetic screw-ups. Enzymes occasionally make errors in the proofreading of DNA, and human scribes occasionally make errors in the proofreading of religious texts. Examples abound in the history of comparative religion. There are multiple passages in the Gospels that contradict one another on such seemingly well-known and agreed upon events as the time and place of Christ's crucifixion. Biblical scholars have noted that the final sections of the Gospels of Saint Mark are stylistically different from the rest of the book, indicating a later addition. For a more dramatic example, take the Islamic suicide bombers who sacrifice themselves in fiery explosions with hopes of landing in the bosoms of 72 beautiful virgins. At a recent conference on Koran interpretation held at the University of Notre

Dame, one scholar suggested that the Arabic word for the 'virgins' promised to martyrs upon arrival in heaven actually refers to 'grapes'. Whether or not this was a misreading of the original, if radical Jihadis started to believe it, the number of terrorist attacks might be reduced.

The Adaptation of Magical Thinkers

After all this talk of religion as genetic by-products and parasitic memes, is there any room left for good old fashioned adaptation? Perhaps. The evolutionary biologist David Sloan Wilson has proposed an adaptationist theory of religion involving a controversial take on Darwinism: group selection. It goes something like this.

In the beginning (prehistoric times), there were multiple isolated groups of humans living in the savannah of Africa and the Near East. Within each group there was a random distribution of magical thinkers (those who were naturally inclined to believe in the afterlife, the power of prayer, and so on) and concrete thinkers (those who were naturally inclined to see the world through the lens of folk physics). By chance, some groups had a higher proportion of magical thinkers than others. Initially, the less practical-minded magical thinkers fared worse than their more rational brethren in terms of survival and reproduction. But very occasionally, in times of great social upheaval or natural catastrophe affecting multiple groups within a geographic region, those groups with a higher concentration of magical thinkers (the hopeful ones) out-competed those groups that did not (the hopeless ones), resulting in a natural selection for magical thinkers in general. Wilson believes that self-sacrifice, which makes no sense from the individual's point of view, can be explained by its contribution to the survival of the group as a whole. The most devout members of every faith have embraced such costly displays and vows of devotion as self-flagellation, self-mutilation, fasting, poverty, and chastity. But what may be disadvantageous at the level of individual selection may actually be adaptive at the group level.

Does this adaptationist argument carry any weight? Let's examine it point by point and find out. I agree with the first premise: there is a natural distribution of magical thinkers. Those roots of thought that function as launching pads for religion are part of human nature. These include the TOMM, agency detectors, innate teleology, recursive logic, language, and so on. They are automatically wired in as soon as the genes for transcription factors, axon guidance, and synaptic plasticity are expressed in our embryonic brains. But we don't all have the same versions of each gene. Some of us carry mutations like FOXP2 and MeCP2 that lead to slightly under-active or hyperactive modules, which, in turn, produce brains that tend to be more or less magically inclined. At the extreme end of the magical thought spectrum are those with temporal lobe personality, schizophrenia, and other types of psychosis. At the opposite end of the bell curve would be people with autism and other concrete thinkers. But most people are distributed somewhere in the middle (Figure 15).

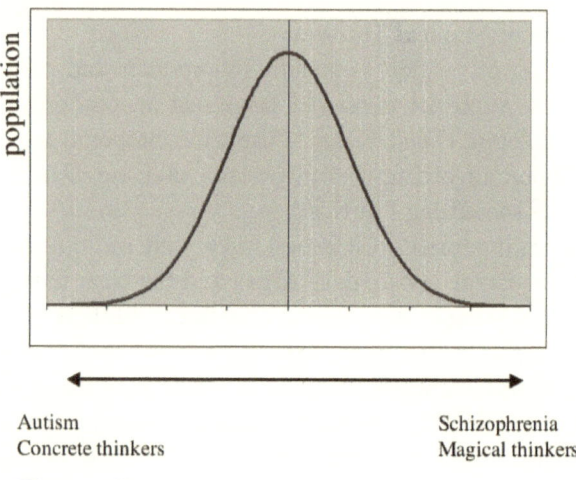

Autism   Schizophrenia
Concrete thinkers   Magical thinkers

Figure 15

I also agree with the second point: the notion that extreme magical thinkers (and also extreme concrete thinkers) are generally less successful socially and reproductively than those who are more 'belief balanced'. We live in a real world that demands real world perception and understanding. Seeing a hidden purpose and meaning behind every little social interaction is just as counterproductive as being mindblind. Why would anyone want to have sex with someone suffering from paranoid delusions? If magical thinking were genetic, natural selection should have weeded it out long ago.

It is with the next point that Wilson's theory runs into difficulty. He believes that human groups behave rather like rival beehives or ant colonies where the members are segregated into specialist castes of workers, warriors, drones, queens, and so on. People who are better folk psychologists (magical thinkers) make up one class while the folk physicists (concrete thinkers) make up another. Each occupies a specific niche in the social hierarchy and contributes something of value to the whole. In this way, most of the individuals of the group benefit more than if each were left to themselves.

Magical thinkers are natural born believers. They believe in the power of prayer to change things for the better. They follow rigorous rules and rituals, and dress in distinctive garb that sets them apart from their fellow nonbelievers. They sacrifice their time, their resources, and sometimes their lives for causes they believe are more important than themselves. They believe they will be justly rewarded in their next life. These beliefs lead to behavior that may be self-sacrificial but gives the rest of the group cohesion and a sense of direction. More importantly, magical thinkers maintain hope in the face of certain doom. They hope that somehow things will get better in the future, if not in this life, than in the one to come. This unswerving hope is transmitted to the community, giving it the power to go on with life where other groups may give up in despair. In the ceaseless competition between rival groups for survival in the midst of limited resources and existential disasters, the hopeful may have an edge.

This line of reasoning appears to make sense in theory, but fails in practice. Human beings are not social insects or cogs in a giant machine. They are individual free agents fully capable of independent thought and decision-making (although many of those decisions are biased by subconscious processes). Numerous political philosophers and social 'scientists' since the mid-nineteenth century have ignored this inconvenient truth, reducing the individual in their cherished models to a mindless particle buffeted by the winds of history. The results have been nothing short of catastrophic. I need not remind readers of the sad legacy of Karl Marx and his henchmen. By subordinating individual human beings to the mechanics of group behavior, Marx thought he had discovered a natural law of social science on par with Newton's laws of planetary motion or Darwin's laws of evolution. But he was terribly mistaken.

Unlike biology, where huge conglomerations of cells, each a potential organism in its own right, acquire emergent identities and function as individual units subject to natural selection, societies generally do not. Social insects, in which individuals have evolved to lose their independence, are a special case. But even there, what seems like group selection is actually a special form of gene selection. Evolutionary biologists call this kin selection, a fascinating topic to which I shall return in the next chapter. In human societies, genes and memes are selected at the level of the individual, because they are much stronger agents than groups could ever be. Group selection could work, in principle, if individuals were weak agents like skin cells or worker ants, just as communism could work, in principle, if people didn't believe they were free, like brainwashed North Koreans or members of a cult. But we are strong, and we believe that we are free (whether we are or not is a separate issue). That is why group selection and communism can never work in fact. Despite the knowledge that tens of millions of people have been murdered in the gulags and collective farms of the former Soviet Union, the 're-education' camps of China, the hellhole of North Korea, and the killing fields of Cambodia, some people on the far left have yet to learn this lesson. Wilson's fatal flaw was to invoke a neo-Marxist line of argument.

Having said all that, I do agree that magical thinkers, through their physical and ritualistic displays, offer the rest of their group cohesion and collective identity. It is also very plausible that habitual wishful thinking does spread hope in desperate situations, imbuing the collective with a sense of optimism. But I don't think that one needs to invoke group selection to explain these things. Dan Dennett comes to the rescue with his updated meme theory. Here it is in his own words:

> 'Memes that foster human group solidarity are particularly fit (as memes) in circumstances in which host survival (and hence host fitness) most directly depends on hosts' joining forces in groups. The success of such meme-infested groups is itself a potent broadcasting device, enhancing outgroup curiosity (and envy) and thus permitting linguistic, ethnic, and geographic boundaries to be more readily penetrated.'
> [Dennett, Breaking the Spell]

The memes that happen to strengthen group identity, such as ritualistic displays, and those that promote group resilience, such as wishful thinking, build groups that further encourage the development of other group-building memes. Because memes are a true second replicator, there is no genetic leash holding them back, as there is with group selection. It does not have to deal with the problem of the individual's strong free agency. According to Dennett, the evolution of organized religion is best explained not by group selection, but by the selection of group-building memes.

Foma
Nothing in this book is true.
Live by the foma that make you brave
And kind and healthy and happy.
Kurt Vonnegut

Imagine there's no heaven, it's easy if you try
No hell below us, above us only sky
Imagine there's no countries, it isn't hard to do
Nothing to kill or die for and no religions too
John Lennon

These are true: there is no consciousness after death, no meaning of life, no cosmic purpose, and no God. Yet all these notions emerged from the interaction of evolved cognitive machinery. All the holy books of every religion were written by men who were sometimes plagued by psychotic delusions. But the contents of these books appeal to the universal human propensity for belief. Religious rituals, taboos, and laws were initially invented by people. But they soon acquired lives of their own as they infected virgin minds and commandeered behavior conducive to social order and authority. Social groups use religion to cement their identity; religion uses social groups to spread its memes.

It is ironic that a phenomenon as divorced from reality as religious belief is, nonetheless fills a gap in the architecture of both the mind and society. For this reason, religion has become a human universal. But harmless untruths that brings health and happiness to so many around the world need not come from religion. There is an innate moral compass inside each of us that predates organized religion and even lies at the core of everything that is good about religion. Many have already found it, especially in the wonderfully secular humanist societies of Denmark and Sweden. Contrary to the common wisdom of many religious conservatives, these atheist Scandinavians are not rampantly immoral, violent, and depraved. Most of them are decent, law-abiding citizens who love their children and cherish the time they spend with their friends and families as much as anyone else. Their rate of violent crime and drug addiction is much lower than that of more religious societies such as the United States. They aren't necessarily hostile to religion, they just don't think about it much. Along with their fellow atheist Dan Dennett, many of them enjoy singing Christmas carols and visiting old churches. They seem to have found a better way outside the magical thought box. All this proves that you don't need God to be good. And conversely, you don't need to be good to find God. But does 'good' mean anything at all in an impersonal universe? What lies beyond good and evil? These are the questions for our last chapter.

Chapter 4

Politics

From the crooked timber of humanity, no truly straight thing can be made.

Immanuel Kant

If I am for myself alone, what am I?
And if I am not for myself, who will be for me?
And if not now, when?

Hillel

The point of Life on Earth is simply to be. We are but a thin coating of scum on the surface of a rusty iron ball. Yet of the millions of species that have evolved and are evolving on this planet, ours is so far the only one to have developed the capacity to reflect upon its condition and look outward beyond its own experience. It's disappointing, really: after all the suffering and struggling, we die wondering what it's all about. Is that all there is?

In this chapter, I will argue that we can live perfectly meaningful lives while accepting wholeheartedly the conclusions of scientific reductionism. Along the way, I will explain how altruism and cooperation evolved from selfish genes, and how this led to a set of innate moral concepts universal to all human societies. I will also try to map our modern political and cultural landscape onto a foundation of innate morality, focusing on the often-misunderstood concepts of *freedom* and *equality*.

Beyond the Selfish Gene

Charles Darwin's theory of natural selection has long been accepted as fact by all serious scientists. But that doesn't mean there weren't bumps along the way. There are many natural phenomena that on the surface seem to violate the famous 'survival of the fittest' principle. Some are by-products of selection for other things. These spandrels include the prevalence of psychiatric disorders such as schizophrenia, autism, and bipolar disorder in high achieving families. It is believed that the genes for high intellect and/or creativity can, in higher doses, lead to mental illness. Others were once beneficial traits which are no longer so, such as the human predilection for fatty foods, a carry over from our ancestors' drive to avoid starvation. Others are fitness indicators, such as the peacock's tail or young men's obsession with motorcycles, which young females of the species find sexually alluring because their brains have evolved to subconsciously and correctly associate these dangerous activities with genes for building strong healthy offspring. Finally, there are independent replicators, which interact with or within other organisms, and whose interests conflict with those of their hosts. These include parasites and memes. The list is long, but none of them actually violate the three central principles of Darwinism: replication, mutation, and selection.

In thinking about human nature and culture, I want to bring up another seeming violation of Darwinism: cooperation. This brings to mind the poetry of John Donne: 'No man is an island, entire of itself; every man is a piece of the continent, a part of the main.' We are social creatures, descended from a long line of social primates going back more than twenty million years in the tropical forests of Africa. In all this time, those individuals who developed brains hardwired to recognize and cooperate with others had a selective advantage over those that did not, and so passed on the genes for those brains and behaviors to their surviving offspring. If we look at the situation from this angle, it is easy to understand the evolution of cooperation.

Human beings are capable of many strange behaviors. Among the strangest is generosity. If we are just Darwinian, utilitarian creatures, motivated to maximize our pleasures and minimize our pains, shouldn't we all be selfish? The purpose of life, from a biological (or indeed a biblical) standpoint is to be fruitful and multiply. Yet most parents are nice to their wayward children, wives often devote themselves to philandering husbands, and which of us has never volunteered a favor to a complete stranger we shall in all likelihood never see again? It is obvious that behaviors like these come with costs in time, money, and reproductive potential. So why are we so nice despite natural selection?

Family Ties

The riddle of altruism was eventually solved using two separate modifications of Darwinism. The first was the theory of *kin selection*, a concept developed by a long line of distinguished English evolutionary biologists, including R. A. Fisher, J. B. S. Haldane, and culminating in the work of William Hamilton in the 1960's. The term itself was coined by John Maynard Smith, and popularized a few years later in a book titled <u>The Selfish Gene</u>, written by Hamilton's colleague from New College, Oxford, Richard Dawkins. It refers to the selfless giving and sharing of food, protection, and affection among members of close and extended families. It is carried to an extreme in some species of social animals such as bees, ants, termites, meerkats, and naked mole rats, members of which literally commit suicide if necessary for the good of the colony. These animals are unique in that all the individuals of a given colony, which may number in the thousands in the case of insects, are siblings. They are related through a common mother, commonly referred to as the queen, and stratified into castes of workers, farmers, soldiers, and other specialists. In humans, such sacrificial acts are not unknown among non-kin, but are usually reserved for members of immediate family.

Haldane knew about the implications of kin selection in the 1950's when he joked that he wouldn't give up his life for his brother, but he would for two brothers, four nephews, or eight cousins. This makes sense when we think about the quantitative benefits to our genes, half of which we share on average with a sibling, a quarter with a nephew, and an eighth with a first cousin. But it was Hamilton who gave the concept mathematical rigor with his equation $rB > C$, where B is the reproductive benefit gained by the recipient of the altruistic act, C is the reproductive cost to the donor of the act, and r is the degree of genetic relatedness of the two individuals. Kin selection makes sense for the survival of one's genes copied in one's relatives.

The difficulty many people have with kin selection is that they believe it debases human nature and undermines free will by reducing our behavior to the cold calculus of genetic survival: we are just prisoners of our genes. This was, and still is, the most common misreading of Hamilton's ideas in Dawkins' The Selfish Gene. Many of us would like to believe that we are generous to our children and relatives simply because *we are good* and it makes us feel good to be good, and not because some piece of deoxyribonucleic acid or some wires in our prefrontal cortex told us to do so. The reaction is understandable. But the truth is that *our genes are selfish*, and it is they that are the units of natural selection. Recall the three principles of Darwinism: replication (reproduction), mutation (change), and selection (competition). Societies, groups, and individuals change and they compete with one another, but do they really replicate? When the British established the North American colonies, did they really create an exact replica of the Olde England? When a couple has a child, is that child an exact replica of her parents? No and no. The only things that truly replicate with a great degree of fidelity (aside from the special case of memes) when individuals reproduce are their genes.

Thus it is at the level of genes, not individuals or societies, that natural selection works. But accepting the selfish gene as the driver of the evolution of our bodies, brains, and minds should not make us discount the importance of our human nature. Genes are not conscious or even subconscious. They make up neither system one nor system two. They are just organic polymers that are good at getting copied and acting as templates for proteins. Because they have no brains, they cannot really care or be selfish or altruistic in the sense that we define those terms. It is more appropriate to say that the *genes behave as though they were selfish*. But those genes do build brains capable of thoughts, emotions, feelings, and behaviors. Our experience lies at this emergent level, not at the level of DNA, genes, and chromosomes. The love we feel for our families is real, even if it was programmed by genes that had no clue what they were doing. An analogy would be the relationship between Great Britain and the United States. Without Britain, there would be no United States. Does that mean that Americans are slaves of the British? Of course not. But Britain remains an important nation, and we don't have to destroy it to preserve the American way of life. In fact, one can argue that an appreciation of all things British can enhance our understanding of our own culture. America can be independent of Great Britain just as our human natures are independent of our selfish genes.

Kin selection works in principle because our bodies are not the only repositories of our genes. Our unique complement of 20,000 genes is normally stuck inside all of our cells and has nowhere else to go. Sex changes all that. The invention of sex by the first eukaryotes some two billion years ago allowed *totipotent germ cells* (eggs and sperm) with complete copies of the parent's genetic profile to act as extra-corporeal surrogates in search of their mates. In asexually reproducing organisms such as bacteria, all daughters are clones of the mother. But in sexual organisms, daughters and sons get half of each parent's genes, a quarter of each grandparent's genes, and so on.

Kin selection requires the ability to distinguish kin from non-kin. This led to the evolution of sensory systems that recognize relatives by their appearance, smell, sounds, and behavior, and calculate the degree of relatedness of each relative in order to make judgments about doling out favors or sacrificing one's life. These systems are quick and instinctive, and carried out by the automatic parts of the nervous system. Humans have the added benefit of the slower but more deliberate system two, which gives us the insight to interpret our genetically programmed instincts. The conscious system is a genuine part of our human nature, but the knowledge that it gives us does not make the instinctive urge any less real. An inherent conflict of the human condition arises from the distinction between the genes that actually program our behavior and the minds that believe that they control it.

Give and Take

Kin selection is not the only way that genes can benefit other copies of themselves. In the early 1970's the renegade American biologist Robert Trivers burst on the scene with the concept of *reciprocal altruism*. An often-cited example occurs in the vampire bat. A bat returns home to her cave engorged after a night of feasting. She is approached by another (unrelated) bat who has been less successful. The sight prompts her to regurgitate some of her blood meal for her begging compatriot. The thankful bat is then expected to reciprocate at some later date. If this occurs, the immediate cost to the donor and her genes is less than its potential future benefit because sharing is cheaper than starving. Zoologists have found that this behavior is relatively common among vampire bats. Reciprocal altruism doesn't even have to involve members of the same species; the exchange can occur between members of widely different species. It explains the relationship between nectar-bearing flowers and bees, sharks and ramoras, clownfish and anemones, and toxoplasma and cats. All symbiotic relationships in which both parties derive cooperative benefits greater than each would be able to gain on its own are, generally speaking, examples of reciprocal altruism. But Trivers was more interested in how this relationship could lead to the evolution of human moral emotions.

It is easy to see how a mutation that programmed an individual to behave cooperatively could lead to collective benefits for the entire group. A society of specialists exchanging the fruits of their labors is superior to one where each man is a jack-of-all-trades and a master of none. This, of course, sums up human progress for the last 10,000 years. But evolution has no foresight. From the Darwinian standpoint, reciprocal altruism is actually quite a difficult thing to achieve. The problem is that it really does pay to cheat. Why would anyone want to cooperate if they could get away without? A generous individual will be worse off when the object of his generosity fails to reciprocate. In a group in which all individuals are programmed to groom one another, a new selfish mutant that accepted grooming but failed to give back would benefit tremendously. This freeloading mutant would enjoy such a selective advantage over its altruistic fellows that his genes would eventually take over the gene pool.

Trivers came to realize that two key components are necessary for reciprocal altruism to work. The first is a way for one to remember who has reciprocated (or cheated) in the past. The second is a dedicated tit-for-tat strategy for punishing cheaters. The remarkable thing is that through the course of evolution, these two components have been fine tuned to such a high degree that cheater detectors are now routinely used to determine if a complete stranger is trustworthy, while potential cheaters are so sophisticated that they routinely deceive even themselves. And both parties have evolved complex emotions which compel them to play the game.

Reciprocation starts with the assumption that if you want me to scratch your back, then I expect you to scratch mine the next time I'm itchy. This is quite unlike the case with close kin, who can expect unconditional back scratching. Reciprocation usually is the rule because we are evolved social animals. Occasionally, we come across a freeloader who doesn't reciprocate. And then what happens? We feel annoyed and cheated. We think he shouldn't be allowed to get away with it. And we often do something about it. Our indignation compels us to rebuke his error: 'make sure it doesn't happen again', or 'I can take my business elsewhere.' If it does happen again, we resort to sterner measures: we tell our friends and associates what a selfish bastard he is, or we report him to the better business bureau, the police, or Uncle Vinnie down at the pool hall. We feel a not unpleasant sense of righteous justice when he is made to suffer pain and humiliation. In the end he will either be forced to play by the rules or be prevented from playing at all.

The tit-for-tat strategy is necessary for reining in freeloaders who would otherwise gum up the reciprocal altruistic strategy that benefits our selfish genes. Without the evolution of vindictiveness and punishment, there could be no cooperation. There is evidence that this is incorporated into our innate mental machinery. Psychologists have devised an experiment called 'the ultimatum game' in which subjects are given an amount of money, say ten dollars, and told to divide it in whichever way they want with another subject. The two can then keep the money. The catch is that the recipient has the power to reject the offer if he feels it is too low, in which case neither gets paid. Rationally, it would make most sense for the donor to give the recipient just one dollar, as any money he gets is better than nothing at all. But in reality, most recipients reject that offer, preferring to punish the donor than to get the dollar. Donors know this, and so most of them share half the amount. However, when subjects were told that their opponent in the ultimatum game was a computer whose behavior could not be predicted, most accepted the computer's offer, however insultingly low. This demonstrates that our impulse to refuse a low offer is based on a desire to punish the person making it by teaching him a painful lesson.

Early versions of cheater detection software were dependent on the memory of past acts of cooperation or defection. As a result, they were easily undermined by new cheater mutations that allowed users to deceive benefactors in more subtle ways. For example, some were able to tell better lies, fake emotions, and otherwise make it seem that they were cooperating when the truth was otherwise. Some developed the talent for advertising and exaggerating their munificence with flowery rhetoric and eloquence to crowds of duped admirers, while others used their wit to charm their way into parasitic relationships. So clever were these mutants, that their victims were often fooled into denying their own predicament, turning away the good advice of their concerned friends and family.

This phenomenon is all too common to this day because it is impossible to completely eliminate freeloader genes. A steady-state equilibrium exists between a majority of cooperators and a minority of sophisticated cheaters rather analogous to the equilibrium between evolving pathogens and responding immune systems, or of plants, herbivores, and carnivores within a balanced ecosystem. But just as in any immune system or ecosystem, the equilibrium is dynamic. Victims are not eternally stupid; they will either go extinct or evolve intelligence. Cheater detectors are constantly evolving to catch, deter, and punish the latest schemer. But the cheaters are always slightly ahead of them, evolving ever more sophisticated ways to get away with yet another a free lunch, which in turn allows the cheater's genes to reproduce and create more such cheaters.

The evolutionary arms race waged between unrelated individuals in cooperative species led to all sorts of interesting adaptations designed to weed out undesirables, such as banishment and the withdrawal of sexual favors. Many animals display these behaviors. But in the human species, with its characteristically oversized brain, the results were particularly bizarre. I will focus on four of them: gossip, moral emotions, self-delusion, and empathy.

The Fruits of Cooperation

The great apes play reciprocal altruism with the currency of grooming (picking off lice and dirt). Those who groom better and more often are treated better in return. In our species, grooming has been replaced by gossip. As was pointed out in the last chapter, the anthropologist Robin Dunbar has discovered that within a given group of species, the average brain size is closely correlated with the average size of the social group. For example, baboons live in bands of a dozen or so members while chimpanzees live in groups of around thirty individuals. Extrapolating to human brains, Dunbar estimates that humans 'naturally' cluster in groups of between 100 to 150 individuals (family, friends, and well known associates). This has been borne out in research into the sizes of people's address books and date planners.

For a group of social primates to cohere, its members must constantly keep in touch, literally. This can be done in groups of a few dozen individuals. But when the numbers exceed a hundred, it becomes almost impossible to use grooming as a method of social bonding. Dunbar believes that the demands of social commitment within progressively more complex groups of individuals forced the evolution of a system of virtual grooming: language. The theory is quite controversial, and probably does not fully explain the evolution of language. But he does rightfully emphasize the importance of a specific use of language that has long been neglected: gossip. Dunbar has done some titillating fieldwork by eavesdropping on the conversation of ordinary people in various situations around the world: commuter trains, amusement parks, airport lounges, supermarkets, and so on. He found that people on average spend *two-thirds* of their speaking time gossiping about other people! The results were quite robust and universal, cutting across age, ethnicity, socioeconomic class, nationality, and perhaps surprisingly, sex. Men tended to gossip less in the company of females, but were just as bad when around other men.

So what is so useful about gossip that most of our speaking time and effort is devoted to it? It doesn't directly help us get from point A to point B, avoid a dangerous predator, or make money. The answer seems to be that it functions to build up one's reputation amongst one's peers. Just like grooming does with chimpanzees, gossiping often and gossiping well (with lots of juicy tidbits about A's sexual indiscretions) raises one's prestige not so much because others will act on the information, but mainly because it functions to bond the gossiper and his listener together. And it is this bond of mutual trust multiplied by 100 or 150 individuals that cements the identity of the tribe.

Moral Emotions

The best way for a gene to get a brain to make more copies of it is to make it *feel* the urge to do so. David Hume was spot on when he said nearly three centuries ago that 'the reasons are the slaves of the passions'. The passions lie buried deep in the limbic centers of the old mammalian brain, and they were around long before the rational, reflective centers of the neocortex evolved around them. This is why the unwise behaviors that allow our genes to get copied into other bodies (such as unsafe sex) feel so good. Likewise, anything that allowed our kin to thrive (such as nepotism) can also be expected to make us feel good, despite our better judgment and the legal system. When it comes to reciprocity, things get more complicated. It is in the best interest of the altruist's genes that the receiver *feels* the compulsion to return the favor. If he felt no such emotion, then his inborn drive to propagate his own genes would trump all, and he would feel the opposing compulsion to cheat instead. That would just lead us back to a gene pool of selfish freeloaders. So it is not enough that the altruists feel the emotion to punishing cheaters; the receivers should also feel the compulsion to cooperate. Trivers introduced the revolutionary notion that thousands of generations of reciprocation led to the evolution of the innate moral emotions found in all human societies today. In addition to the anger and vindictiveness felt by the cheated altruist, there is also gratitude, guilt, sympathy, affection, and love, felt by benefactor and beneficiary alike.

Gratitude is the feeling that compels the recipient to express thanks to his benefactor and makes him want to pay back his debt. Guilt is the feeling of pain felt by the recipient who has cheated his benefactor and makes him want to redress past wrongs. Sympathy is the feeling one gets for someone who could use a helping hand; it is what usually sets off the cycle of reciprocation. Love and affection are the feelings we normally have for those whose genes we share (our children, siblings, and other relatives) and for our mates, who, of course, make a direct contribution to our offspring. But sometimes we also feel love for non-kin with whom the cycle of reciprocation has reached a level of trust and expectation that makes the relationship as beneficial as anything we can have with our family. These moral emotions are innate and universal, meaning that they evolved over thousands of cycles of natural selection, are coded into our DNA, and expressed in our brain tissue. The moral emotions make our brains feel the need to cooperate, spread gossip, punish cheaters, repay debts, avoid punishment, and love those who love us back. But even they are not enough to weed out the most recalcitrant cheaters.

Self Deception

Unfortunately, it does pay to cheat if you can get away with it. The problem is that the art of pathological lying is actually quite difficult to perfect. Try it sometime. Our facial expressions, exquisitely sensitive to the moral emotion of guilt, give us away. Evolution has solved this conundrum with a brilliant adaptation: why not believe your own lies? The Machiavellian arms race between cooperators and defectors has reached its twisted pinnacle with the evolution of self-deception.

Psychologists have done many experiments that support the existence of self-serving biases. When a random sample of people are asked to rank their ability or intelligence compared with their peers, a majority of them consistently rate themselves 'above average'. When test subjects are asked to flip a coin to decide whether they or their (hidden) partners are to get a prize, ninety percent of them claim that they 'won' the coin toss. When people are asked how much money others would donate to a charity event, they are fairly accurate, but when asked how much they themselves would give, they consistently overestimate the amount. And when asked about their behavior later, they rationalize some excuse: 'I've always been told I was above average', 'I really meant tails I don't lose', or 'I would have given more, but I just gave to another charity not too long ago.'

Self-deception and hypocrisy are so prevalent because they are the results of the interaction between innate defense mechanisms and the rest of our mental architecture. It is natural for system one to be biased towards itself; it was programmed to be selfish by the genes that made it. In contrast, system two evolved under the selective pressure of a social environment that values cooperation and reciprocity. So the interpreter has learned to put a positive spin on subconsciously driven selfish behavior. It rationalizes our self-serving biases to make it seem that we are more benevolent than we really are. The distressing part is that we actually believe this deception. We can't help it; *the interpreter simply is our conscious self.* We are so easily fooled because the source and the target of the deception are one and the same.

In certain cases of brain damage, the interpreter's capacity to confabulate seems boundless. Patients with left hemineglect resulting from a stroke to the right parietal lobe will sometimes say that objects on the left side are 'not very interesting', rather than admit that they can't see them. Patients suffering from Capgras' syndrome, caused by the disconnection of the amygdala from the prefrontal areas, claim that familiar people are impostors, rather than admit that they don't seem familiar. Patients suffering from Alzheimer's dementia caused by the degeneration of hippocampal neurons often downplay their mistakes with excuses – they were never very good with names, or they don't like Democrats – rather than admit that they can't remember who the president is. These are all examples of the left hemisphere interpreter gone amok. In neurologically intact individuals, the phenomenon is less extreme, but no less real. It was naturally selected because, as every criminal psychologist knows, the best way to deceive someone else is to believe your own lies.

Self-serving biases are the basis for hypocrisy and self-righteousness. The interpreter's self-serving rationalizations blind us to our baser motives while convincing us of our benevolence. The flip side of this is the belief that others are inferior, immoral, or just plain evil. The social psychologist Roy Baumeister believes that there are four root causes of violence and cruelty: greed/ambition, sadism, high self-esteem, and moral idealism. Of those, the last two are the biggest factors. This may seem surprising, but think about how much violence is caused by young men who feel their reputations have been threatened by some real or imagined rival. And on a larger scale, think about how many feuds and wars have been stoked by the 'bad guys' on the other side who always seem to be in the wrong. The world would be a much more peaceful place if we were not so quick to find faults in others, while ignoring bigger ones in ourselves. But, as we shall see later, this inequality born of the conflict between autonomy and cooperation leads as often to love as it does to violence, and lies at the core of human politics.

Mimicry, Empathy, and the Mirror Neuron
Have you ever noticed that when someone speaks to you in a foreign accent, you find yourself inadvertently imitating his accent, even if you don't know his language? Do you smile back when someone smiles at you, choke up when you see someone in tears, and wince when someone stubs their toe? Have

you ever waved your arms in unison with a thousand others at a rock concert and felt one with the crowd? These are examples of mimicry, another human universal inherited from our mammalian ancestors. The propensity to imitate starts when a baby is a few months old and persists throughout life. Those afflicted by dementia or brain damage sometimes exhibit an overabundance of it. On the other hand, people pathologically unable to imitate others suffer social isolation and emotional distress.

As the saying goes, imitation is the highest form of flattery. We tend to imitate people we like, and we like people who imitate us. We go out of our way to engage in activities that involve synchronized motion, such as dancing, karaoke, and prayer. We subconsciously copy our friends' gestures in conversation. It simply feels good to imitate. Evolutionary psychology teaches us that pleasurable things usually have a selective advantage. Social scientists have long suspected that mimicry and *social contagion* function as an instinctive device designed to bond individuals to the group. Neuroscientists have now proven them right.

In 1991, Giacomo Rizzolati and his colleagues at the University of Parma were investigating the properties of motor neurons in macaque monkeys. They had hooked up their subjects to electrodes that recorded the activities of individual cells in the motor cortex. Each motor neuron codes for a specific movement. So it was not surprising that these neurons fired when the creatures grabbed a peanut and moved it in a specific direction. But then the Italian team discovered something extraordinary: a graduate student brought in a gelato and moved it towards her lips. The electrode attached to the motor neuron fired, even though the monkey was doing nothing other than looking at the hungry graduate student. Rizzolati's team soon found many such neurons scattered throughout several nearby regions of the monkey's brain, each corresponding to an action made by the animal, as expected, *and* to the observation of a similar movement made by someone else, which was totally unexpected. The Italians had discovered what soon came to be known as the *mirror neuron*.

The finding was so pregnant with potential not just for cognitive neuroscience, but for social science in general, that in the year 2000, V. S. Ramachandran was inspired to predict that 'mirror neurons will do for psychology what DNA did for biology' in an essay for John Brockman's Edge Page titled "Mirror Neurons and Imitation Learning as the Driving Force Behind 'the Great Leap Forward' in Human Evolution." Hyperbole aside, the implications of mirror neurons for understanding the neural basis of intention, empathy, Theory of Mind, language, learning and learnability, cultural evolution, and even self-consciousness are truly exciting.

These cells are no different from garden-variety cortical neurons in their anatomy and physiology. The distinction lies in the organization of their networks. In the monkey, they are found in the inferior parietal and ventral premotor cortex, the parts of the brain that specialize in the analysis of perceived motion and in the higher-order planning of movements, respectively. These areas correspond to the later stages of the dorsal stream, which, you will recall, is the 'where' or 'how to' pathway. Because it is unethical to stick needles into the brains of healthy volunteers, the existence of mirror neurons has not yet been directly confirmed in humans. But there is a wealth of indirect evidence from studies using EEG, MEG, fMRI, and PET scans indicating that we have them as well. In humans, brain areas with mirror-like properties have been localized to parts of the frontal cortex (including the insula) in addition to the inferior parietal/premotor areas. All of these places light up both when subjects see/experience something and when they see/imagine someone else experiencing the same thing. These regions receive input from the fusiform face processing area and parts of the superior temporal lobe specializing in the perception of biological motion, and send output to the prefrontal cortex where conscious judgments are carried out.

In the wake of Rizzolati's discovery, psychologists and philosophers of mind came up with a theory explaining how people come to understand each other's behaviors and emotions. The *simulation theory* or *direct-matching hypothesis* builds on William James's idea that people comprehend their own intentions after monitoring their actions, rather than the other way around. Bertrand Russell was on right track when he asked, 'how do I know what I think until I see what I say?' Volitional acts are instigated by subconscious mechanisms that are consciously interpreted only after the fact. Similarly, the argument goes, people may comprehend others' intentions after mirroring the observed actions in their own minds and then deducing backwards from that simulation. The direct-matching hypothesis provides an essential link not only between action and intention but also between the representations of self and of others. The cognitive psychologists Sarah-Jayne Blakemore and Jean Decety summarize this notion nicely:

> 'When we observe another person's actions…the observed sensory consequences (of another person's actions) would be mapped onto stored sensory predictions (of the sensory consequences of one's own actions). These stored representations could then be used to estimate the motor commands and intentions that would normally precede such an action. This could be achieved by automatically and unconsciously simulating the observed action and estimating

what our own intentions would be if we produced the same action within the same context.

By simulating another person's actions and mapping them onto stored representations of our own motor commands and their consequences... it might be possible to estimate the observed person's internal states, which cannot be read directly from their movements. This simulating system could also provide information from which predictions about the person's future actions could be made.' [From the Perception of Action to the Understanding of Intention, Nature Reviews Neuroscience, Aug 2001]

Sensory-motor linkage is not the only thing that can be mirrored. When subjects are exposed to offensive odors while inside an fMRI scanner, their insulae, along with their olfactory areas, are usually activated as expected. Recall that this is a part of the brain that processes incoming negative emotions. But when they are shown pictures of other people with disgusted expressions on their faces, the insula lights up once again. When people are shown images of someone holding a pair of scissors, there is activity in parts of the temporal cortex involved in tool perception. But when they see scissors about to cut someone's finger, the anterior cingulate cortex, the part of the brain that is normally activated by the perception on one's own pain, lights up as well. Experiments like these indicate that there are multiple mirror systems scattered throughout the human brain that allow us to detect and simulate not just the actions of others, but their perceptions and emotions as well. We are endowed with motion and emotion detectors that were designed by natural selection to allow us to live vicariously through the experiences of those close to us. Even if we cannot do or see or feel what the other is doing, seeing, or feeling, our brains come loaded with virtual reality software that can tell us what it is like. We call this empathy. It is a trick that builds bonds and aids the process of reciprocation between individuals who would not otherwise be compelled to cooperate.

It should be noted, however, that empathy is not the same as identity. We know when we are pretending. Just as a dream, no matter how vivid, is never as richly textured as reality, the simulated experiences we get from our mirror systems are not as intense as if we ourselves had just scored the winning touchdown, aborted the baby, won the lottery, or stubbed a toe. I can empathize with your pleasures and pains, but I can't actually feel them like you do. When I see Roger Federer play tennis, I can picture myself making his forehand passing shot in my mind's eye and in my mind's body, but of course it's not the same. There are good reasons and mechanisms for this. We need to know the difference between ourselves and others. As social as we are, we are not clones, but rather individuals who respect our boundaries and expect others to do the same. If empathy melted into identity, those borders would crumble. We might as well be the same organism. Our selfish genes have seen to it that the self-systems are segregated from the mirror systems in the brain. Self-generated motions are processed partly in the cerebellum, and take a more roundabout course to the prefrontal cortex than observed motions.

This is what usually happens. But as is so often the case in neuroscience, there are exceptions. Normally, people cannot tickle themselves, no matter how ticklish they may be. This is because the neural patterns corresponding to the perception of self-generated actions go through two channels, one of which passes through the cerebellum. The cerebellular pathway takes a bit longer, and this delay acts as a feedback brake on the final perception of the ticklish feeling. Perceptions of external stimuli do not involve the cerebellum and consequently there is no inhibition of the tickle. However, there is some anecdotal evidence that some individuals suffering from psychosis are able to tickle themselves, possibly due to a down-regulation of the cerebellum. Indeed, the very hallmark of schizophrenia is the inability to distinguish perceptions and feelings generated from outside (external reality) from those that they conjure up in their own minds. It is unclear if schizophrenia involves up-regulation of mirror neurons directly, but the inability to distinguish self from other lies at its core. At the opposite extreme are the autistic disorders, which are characterized, among other things, by the inability to empathize with others. Autistics, as I mentioned earlier, are 'mindblind' because they have a difficult time imagining what it is like to be in someone else's shoes. Researchers like Antonio Damasio and Ramachandran have recently discovered that the mirror neuron-rich regions of the brain are underactive in autistic subjects.

Self and Other
So what do mirror neurons have to do with culture and consciousness? Ramachandran, Nicholas Humphrey, and others have speculated that the core function of the mirror network is a computational transformation of one kind of representation into another, for example, perceptual input into motor output. In addition to its original purpose of understanding others, it has evolved new uses. One is speech, which involves linking a sound or 'phoneme' to a corresponding movement of the lip and tongue. This may initially have been facilitated by a type of mirror neuron. Another is metaphor, which requires the ability to link sensory, motor, emotional, and analytical concepts together into one nugget: 'I'll be sure to get right on top of it' or 'I'm feeling

high as a kite'. Cross-modal linkage like this is the mirror neuron's specialty. A third mirror spin-off was the discovery of imitation learning. Monkey-see, monkey-do doesn't just make more empathetic monkeys, it makes smarter ones. Combined with language, memory, and metaphoric thought, imitation allows teachers to pass on acquired know-how to pupils without having them learn through trial and error. Once in place, imitation learning was so efficient and economical that our ancestors could accumulate useful knowledge over a lifetime and transmit it to others. This formed the basis of human cultural evolution through a second replicator. About 100,000 years ago, the mirror neuron gave birth to the first meme.

Perhaps the most remarkable application of the mirror neuron is self-discovery. Ramachandran introduced this radical idea in a pair of speculative essays written for John Brockman's online salon, Edge.org in 2006 and 2007. It goes something like this. Mirror neurons were originally used for predicting the actions of others by simulating their observed behaviors in one's own motor circuits. A similar trick was later used to read the intentions of others by simulating their facial expressions in one's own limbic circuits. In this way, motor understanding led to mind reading, empathy, and Theory of Mind. But it didn't stop there. The human brain is equipped with body maps in the inferior parietal lobe of both hemispheres. The body maps allow you to imagine or visualize your body in space as if you were a third person. This is adaptive for situations that require preparing the body to squeeze through or maneuver in tight spaces, for example. According to Ramachandran, it is no coincidence that these areas are also known to have a high concentration of mirror circuits.

The mirror neurons that allow understanding of others were then co-opted, via the self-body maps in the parietal lobes, to *reflect back* on the self. In Ramachandran's words:

> 'I suggest that self-awareness is simply using mirror neurons
> for "looking at myself as if someone else is looking at me"
> (the word "me" encompassing some of my brain processes, as
> well). The mirror neuron mechanism — the same algorithm
> — that originally evolved to help you adopt another's point
> of view was turned inward to look at your own self. This,
> in essence, is the basis of things like "introspection". It may
> not be coincidental that we use phrases like "self conscious"
> when you really mean that you are conscious of others being
> conscious of you. Or say "I am reflecting" when you mean
> you are aware of yourself thinking. In other words the ability
> to turn inward to introspect or reflect may be a sort of

metaphorical extension of the mirror neuron's ability to read others' minds. It is often tacitly assumed that the uniquely human ability to construct a "theory of other minds" or "TOM" (seeing the world from the other's point of view; "mind reading", figuring out what someone is up to, etc.) must come after an already pre-existing sense of self. I am arguing that the exact opposite is true; the TOM evolved first in response to social needs and then later, as an unexpected bonus, came the ability to introspect on your own thoughts and intentions. ['The Brain in the Vat', <u>Edge.org</u>, Jan 12, 2006]

If Ramachandran is right, *self-consciousness* and the very notion of *self* are illusions experienced by the talkative interpreter in the left hemisphere, and also by the mute right hemisphere, in response to self-referential mirror neuron activity in the inferior parietal lobe. But they are very adaptive illusions insomuch as they *directly* facilitate getting our genes replicated into the next generation. On the other hand, the knowledge of and the empathetic feeling towards others are illusions experienced in response to mirror neuron activity in the insula, anterior cingulate, and other limbic regions. They, too, are adaptive illusions in that they get our genes *indirectly* replicated via kin selection and reciprocal altruism. Autonomy and cooperation are simply two different strategies employed by our selfish genes throughout millions of years of evolution. Both strategies start with the mirror neuron.

The Origin of Conflict
To be human is to suffer and to know that we suffer. As the song goes, 'life's a bitch, and then you die'. One would think that this knowledge alone would be enough to get us to come together and love one another right now. All you need is peace, love, and understanding (and some good weed). Catch my drift? The central teaching point of the *Upanishads* and the *Dhammapada*, those wise and ancient texts of Hinduism and its offshoot Buddhism, is that you suffer because you are self-conscious. Somewhere on the road from creation, you found your self, but lost the rest of the universe in the process. Your selfish cares matter only to you, and yet you feel they are the center of all things. The cares of all the others – which are just as important to each of them as yours are to you – seem negligible. Why should you care about total strangers who don't give a damn about you? Therein lies the suffering of humankind.

The Asian mystics offer a solution: ignore the self. Someone who annihilates the illusion of self-awareness will appreciate and embrace the rest of the universe (specifically other people) as a result. Only by destroying your petty attachment to your self can you one open up to others. Meditation, medication, and distraction are the three most common ways of doing this. This philosophy is appealing to many, and the techniques of renunciation do work up to a point, but they are not enough. Even if the entire world converted to Hinduism, Buddhism, and Taoism, there would still be suffering, hatred, and violence. India and China are not exactly paradigms of utopia. I believe that the Eastern philosophies are flawed. We cannot simply renounce the self because the self is woven into the very fabric of our evolved human nature. We can choose to ignore it for a while, but it will always come back with a vengeance.

The only way to completely overcome selfishness is to give up being conscious altogether and meld our minds with the 'mainframe'. But this would require that we all have identical thoughts. Because we are not clones (even identical twins are not psychologically identical), each of us has evolved to perceive the world from our unique self-centered perspective. And when we see ourselves from that perspective, we always appear more important than others.

There is another way. It involves accepting our selfish selves and advocating for them in the bustling marketplace of other selves. You exist. So do others exist. Learn to compromise. Life is meant to be lived; you were created by your parents' selfish desires for each other. To crawl into a cave or an opium den and meditate or medicate your precious time away is not the answer. The selfish genes created a wonderful tool that comes as part of our standard equipment: the mirror neuron system that acts as a bridge between self-understanding and the understanding of others. Learn how to use it! How we choose to use this tool is the subject of morality.

The origin of conflict comes from the double-edged sword of autonomy and cooperation. We want to help our family and friends, but when push comes to shove most of us think of ourselves first. We have to calibrate the love and attention we devote to ourselves and to others. And it is not an equal distribution. The rules of kin selection dictate that we love our children more than our parents, our parents more than our grandparents, and our grandparents more than our in-laws. The rules of reciprocal altruism dictate that we feel more sympathetic to our friends than to our neighbors, our neighbors more than our fellow countrymen, and our countrymen more than some strangers in Haiti. The further we venture out from the center of our self-consciousness and self-interest, the less intense our willingness and ability to empathize. As social animals, we cannot afford to ignore others, but treating everyone with equal care and affection would necessarily mean that those close to us are not close at all.

The Genealogy of Morals

Morality does not lie in the stars. But neither is it a social construct, an arbitrary by-product of cultural history. Our moral sense comes from somewhere in between: it is written in our genes. Now, at the dawn of the twenty-first century, social science, neuroscience, and gene science are finally teaming up to uncover the natural architecture of the human moral sense. It is a quest with roots as deep as philosophy itself. Speculations on the foundations of ethics and morality were central to the works of Plato and Aristotle, the Judeo-Christian prophets, and the ancient Indian mystics thousands of years before the invention of functional magnetic resonance brain scanners and DNA sequencers. Ancient armchair philosophers came up with some profound insights about people's beliefs, behaviors, and conflicts, and used them to make sage recommendations about how life ought to be lived that are still very relevant to us today. But because they knew nothing about the brain or genes, they could only guess as to why people arrive at the convictions they do about right and wrong. Modern science is now putting flesh on those old concepts.

Many people are uncomfortable with the new science of morality and what it may discover. Conservatives fear that taking right and wrong away from God will lead to moral relativism, cultural decadence, and the destruction of cherished traditions. Liberals fear that reducing right and wrong to genetic and neurological mechanisms threatens our free will, undermines human dignity, and denies our faith in self-improvement. Such fears are understandable, but unfounded. Yes, science does discourage the belief in a supernatural god, and it does reduce complex phenomena like morality to more manageable chunks like brain circuits and gene expression patterns. But this viewpoint does nothing to undermine age-old traditions and particular ethical beliefs, nor does it limit the range of human behaviors, thoughts, and laudable efforts at self-improvement. Science cannot tell us what to do, it simply tells us why things are the way they are; it is up to us to figure out how our lives ought to be lived.

The psychologist Donald Brown has compiled a list of human universals: behavioral and linguistic traits that are found in all human cultures without exception. They include, among others, belief in the supernatural, conflict, cooperation, empathy, in-group/out-group distinction, self/other, good/evil, status, dominance/submission, and the concept of fairness. The fact that these traits are common even to aboriginal cultures that had no contact with each other or with outside world before the twentieth century, such as the *Dani* people of highland New Guinea and the *Yanomamö* of deep Amazonia, makes it quite plausible that they evolved through gene-based natural and/or sexual selection rather than through common cultural development. To prove this, we would first need to demonstrate heritability and then, if possible, find the genes responsible for the traits. We know from twin studies that intelligence, personality, and language skills are highly heritable, and scientists have even identified some of the genes involved. These would make ideal models for research on the moral universals.

Perhaps the most important discovery in social neuroscience over the last two decades was the concept of *innate morality*. When social scientists noticed that elements of classical ethics such as fairness and empathy were on the list of human universals, they began to wonder how those entities interacted with one another to create an inborn sense of moral order. The evidence is now quite compelling that this is achieved by genetic programs expressed in each child's developing brain. These programs were the result of evolutionary tinkering over thousands of cycles of courtship and reproduction in that child's ancestors. Of course, some things are learned. What I want to emphasize here is that learning occurs *on top of* preexisting moral settings that were programmed into our neural hardware by the brain-building genes we inherited from our parents.

Psychologist Jonathan Haidt defines morality as 'any system of interlocking values, practices, institutions, and psychological mechanisms that work together to suppress or regulate selfishness and make social life possible'. He came to this conclusion after living with a traditional family as a graduate student in the exotic south Indian temple city of *Bhubaneswar*. It was there that Haidt came to realize that the point of morality is not to facilitate individual striving and self-expression, but rather to give people a framework within which to survive and flourish in the company of others. To this end, Haidt and the anthropologist Richard Shweder have identified five core elements of the innate moral sense: *harm/care, fairness/reciprocity, community/loyalty, authority/respect, and purity/sanctity*. Not only are all five common to all ethnicities and cultures ever studied, but they are also routinely exhibited by young children and, at least in the case of the first four, some social animals as well. These five elements form a 'periodic table of morality' that can be combined with one another to create the complexity of human social intercourse. Let's examine each one.

Fairness
Fairness comes from reciprocal altruism. At its core are the natural human tendencies to be sympathetic to those in need, expect future paybacks from grateful recipients, and feel righteous anger towards those who cheat us. As we saw earlier, these emotions are simply innate functions of neural circuits that

have evolved in animals selected to reproduce in highly social environments. They are designed to be deployed in situations in which generous actions now may reap benefits later. These emotions are effortless and subconscious. Rhesus macaque monkeys have them. In our species, the tit-for-tat strategy and cheater punishment algorithms have been coupled to language, gossip, and a greatly expanded working memory, and modified by further rounds of selective competition between cheaters and cheater detectors. The result is a cognitive module or 'sphere' that straddles both the subconscious and conscious levels of the mind, motivating us to both reciprocate and to rationalize our reciprocation.

The Western legal tradition is largely based on concepts of dispassionate justice and inherent rights, implying that people are naturally rational creatures whose decisions are guided by conscious knowledge of universal right and wrong. That is an erroneous assumption. Functional MRI scans of volunteers playing the ultimatum game reveal that the insula and other parts of the limbic system are among the first parts of the brain to light up when a player gets a bad deal. This happens a split second before he is even aware of the emotion. But the limbic activation is often enough to set up a retaliatory response that the cortex may not be able to stop once in motion.

Consciousness is only the tip of our mental iceberg, and even that fragment is not totally rational. The illusion of the all-powerful interpreter can lead to some uncomfortable rationalizations. For example, many would agree that aging former Nazi concentration camp guards living under false identities should be rounded up and sent to prison for the rest of their remaining years. When questioned why, some may deny vindictiveness but claim that justice should be doled out for the sake of deterrence. Yet these old men are now highly unlikely to hurt any one else, and punishing them will only add to public spending without making another genocide less likely. Who benefits? The dead will remain dead, the war criminals and their families will suffer, further crimes will not be prevented, and the public will have to foot the bill for trials and incarcerations. The only benefit is a smug sense of collective self-righteousness that someone bad didn't get away with his crime. The satisfaction is genuine, but its rationalization is not.

There are no such things as universal good and evil, or rights and wrongs independent of human nature. There are common agreements on moral values based on millions of years of evolution of mirror neurons, dopamine synapses, and limbic-frontal circuits. The abstract concepts of fairness and justice are two of them. But the minute details that constitute what is fair and what is just cannot be coded by individual genes; they are too arbitrary for that level of reduction. How much tip one should leave the waiter, how long to wait before sending a thank you card, how much punishment fits the crime; these vary from culture to culture. The fine-tuning happens at the level of culture.

Reciprocal justice is the basis for many moral systems worldwide. It is the golden rule at the center of Judeo-Christian ethics. This sounds good, but could a society based solely on conceptions of reciprocation and punishment really work? Only if people were basically generous, trusting, and unbiased in their dealings with family, friends, acquaintances, and strangers. But there are three reasons that people are not like that.

First, people are not all the same. Different individuals have a wide range of personalities and temperaments caused by natural gene variants that predispose them to be more or less generous, trusting, or biased, on average, than others. Second, because of the effects of kin selection on human psychology, it is natural for us to be more sympathetic, generous, and trusting of our close family members than of our friends, our friends than casual acquaintances, and acquaintances than complete strangers. Third, we are loaded with self-serving biases that work to magnify the shortcomings of others, while minimizing our own faults. We perceive our motives and actions through rose-colored glasses, and rationalize away our mistakes and prejudices, but we remove those glasses when scrutinizing the motives and mistakes of others. Because of these three reasons, it is impossible for people to be completely fair in practice. The golden rule and any social system based solely on it is wishful fantasy. Fairness and justice are not the basis of real communities, although they are essential to protect individual autonomy.

Loyalty

Consider the following scenario, concocted by Jonathan Haidt. A woman cleaning her house happens to come upon an old and tattered American flag in the closet. She doesn't want it any more, so she cuts it up and uses it to wipe her bathroom floor. Is she wrong to do this, and if so, why? When Haidt presented this question to students around the country in an online survey, most responded negatively to the woman's actions. Even though no one is harmed, no national interests are threatened, and the incident happens in private in the woman's home with her personal property, it still makes people uneasy. This scenario illuminates a second moral sphere quite distinct from fairness. People are naturally inclined to congregate in groups, including family, friends, coworkers, fellow sports fans and hobbyists, and most broadly, countrymen. Whether we consciously intend to or not, we seek out and find comfort in the company of those who share our genes, interests, opinions, prejudices, grievances, talents, handicaps, faith, skepticism, sexual orientation, ethnicity, and racial characteristics. We like those who like us, but we also like those who are like us. This forms the basis for community.

Community, or the notion of loyalty to one's group, is a second innate moral sphere. It is derived from kin selection rather than from reciprocal altruism. As I discussed earlier, people are hardwired to discriminate relatives, with whom they share their genes, from strangers. Unlike reciprocal altruism, where payback under threat of punishment is the norm, people commonly lavish favors and gifts on family members without any expectation of return. This is because in a sense, the happiness and success of a family member is an extension of one's own. In the course of cultural evolution, humans learned to congregate into larger and larger groups where most others were not kin. Reciprocation became the dominant strategy at these levels, but the kinship-detectors were still active and were broadened to detect non-kin as the circle of inclusiveness expanded. We can displace our innate loyalty from family to those who simply share some of our characteristics. We support these pseudo-kin with donations and good deeds, defend them from mutual enemies, and idealize them with kinship names like 'band of brothers'. The instinctive drive to identify with large groups has made communities, clubs, and nations possible. The price is the loss of fairness towards those who are different.

Empathy

A third moral sphere involves the innate revulsion at the sight of another's pain. The mirror neurons in the limbic system allow us to empathize with others' suffering and motivate our frontal lobes to alleviate it as if we were suffering ourselves. This sentiment is echoed in the ethical codes of all cultures throughout human history from the Oath of Hippocrates to the Constitution of the United States. Only recently, however, has it been subjected to neuroscientific inquiry.

In the 1950's, a young British moral philosopher named Philippa Foot invented what later became known as the 'trolley problem'. Basically it goes like this. Imagine a runaway trolley car speeding down the tracks towards five unsuspecting workers. You are standing at a fork with access to a switch that will divert the trolley onto an adjacent spur. The problem is that there happens to be another worker on that spur. Doing nothing will kill five people; pulling the switch will save them, but lead to the death of one. What would you do? Most people respond quite reasonably that they would pull the switch. Some may even argue that one is morally obligated to pull the switch. In the classical utilitarian tradition, it is better to sacrifice the few to save the many. One death is bad, but it's worth a net gain of four saved lives. The rational mind chooses the utilitarian approach because it yields the fairest outcome. But let's make things more complicated.

In one variation of the trolley problem, you are standing on a bridge over the errant trolley on its way to crushing five hapless workers. There is no switch to pull, but there is an unsuspecting very fat man standing next to you. By pushing the man off the bridge directly onto the tracks below, you will stop the trolley from killing the five men, but he himself would be killed as a result. Most balk at that solution. Even with the realization that the end result is the same, the act of manhandling an innocent bystander somehow seems different from simply pulling a switch. The evolutionary biologist Marc Hauser and his colleagues conducted an internet-based experiment in which over 200,000 participants from over a hundred countries responded to a questionnaire about these and related trolley scenarios. The respondents represented a cross-section of humanity: men and women of all ages, races, ethnicities, religions, and educational and socioeconomic backgrounds. The results were consistent. According to the survey, most people say that they would pull a switch that would cause someone's death, but they would not willingly push a person to his death to achieve the same result. It should be noted, of course, that it is impossible to determine what people would actually do in these situations.

These results make some very interesting assumptions about the morality of harm. First, its universality across human populations is highly suggestive of innateness. Like intuitive grammar, folk physics, or the Theory of Mind, the moral sense is an instinct wired into the developing brain. Second, it is more emotional than rational. The German philosopher Immanuel Kant tried to formulate an axiom as to why people should not hurt others. The best he could do was the *categorical imperative* that one should not use another's life as a means to an end. This has been applied to explain the different responses to the trolley problem. In the first case, it is permissible to pull a switch because one is using a mechanical object to save the others; the victim is simply collateral damage. In the second case, it is not permissible to push the fat man off the bridge because that would be the active use of a human being to achieve a goal. Kant may be regarded as a great philosopher, but he seems to have been wrestling with a concept that he found difficult to rationalize. In responding to the threat of moral relativism poised by his formidable British rival David Hume, Kant was determined to carve morality into the solid bedrock of reason. But morality is written neither in reasons nor in stones. The Kantian moral imperative seems artificial and ad hoc because he got it backwards. The reason that we don't want to harm others is not because we know that lives shouldn't be used as tools; rather, we choose not to use lives as tools because we feel bad about harming others. It is the feeling that needs explaining, not the behavior that comes from it.

The solution to 'trolleyology' finally came not from moral philosophy but from social and affective neuroscience. In 2004, the cognitive neuroscientists Joshua Green and Jonathan Cohen of Princeton University conducted a series of experiments in which volunteers were asked to ponder the variations of the trolley problem while their brains were being imaged by fMRI scanners. They found that in the first case (pulling the switch), the medial prefrontal areas were most active. Recall that this is the part of the brain that makes 'rational' decisions. In the fat man variation, the limbic areas and the anterior cingulate cortex were also activated. These are the centers of emotions and conflict resolution. It appears that in situations that involve direct harm, such as physically manhandling another person, a much stronger emotional reaction is elicited in the brain. The mechanism is probably the mirror neuron networks in the limbic system that allow us to feel another's pain. What is unique about the trolley problem is that two distinct brain systems are recruited which conflict with each other. The rational, utilitarian brain argues that it is permissible to kill one to save many. The emotional, empathetic brain recoils from killing anyone, even if many will die. Kant believed that it was reasonable not to want to hurt another, but it is not. When faced with life and death decisions, we rely more on passion than on reason. This is why most of us would probably leave the fat man alone, as the two of us watch with morbid fascination the trolley plowing over those poor workmen.

Our passions can move us to care as much as they can push us to harm. Our mirror neurons make it almost as difficult for us to hurt others as it is to hurt ourselves. But the system only works when we can visualize ourselves in the act of causing direct harm. It does not apply to pushing switches, pulling triggers, turning knobs, barking out nuclear codes, opening bomb bay doors, or signing death warrants. The limbic system can only function as a brake when it is directly engaged. The problem with modern technology is that there are too many ways to separate our rational decision-making process from our emotional safety valve. Society itself has become an impersonal, military-industrial complex. The limbic system, which is normally able to override the prefrontal cortex, doesn't even get recruited.

This brings me to gun control. It has not escaped my attention that the reason why the homicide rate is so much higher in the United States than in any other industrialized nation is our wildly permissive gun laws. Americans are not more or less moral than anyone else. Their capacity for empathy is as well developed as that of the British, the Canadians, the Germans, and the Japanese. Yet many more people die violent deaths here than in those other countries. The problem is not so much cultural, but legal. Not only is it much easier to pull a trigger than to choke, stab, or bludgeon someone to death, but also less repugnant in the perpetrator's mind. The National Rifle Association likes to say, 'guns don't kill people, people kill people'. But removing all guns would make it much more difficult for people to kill people. Only a small minority of hardened criminals and psychopaths would be willing and able to kill with their bare hands. Most people who commit murder with a firearm probably do so out of convenience and impulse, not because they are natural born killers. I'm sure most of them profoundly regret their foolish action the next morning. We don't have to change human nature; we just have to change the laws. How many more Columbines and Virginia Techs will it take for this to happen? How many more innocent lives need to be wasted for Americans to come to their senses? I am embarrassed for my country. If only stricter gun laws were legislated, enforced, and adjudicated, the natural deterrent of the limbic system would be better able to keep us in line. For this reason alone, I urge that Congress and President Obama pass a comprehensive ban on the possession of all personal handguns effectively immediately.

Interestingly, the moral sphere of harm/care often undermines fairness. The fair and just thing to do is to treat everyone with equal care regardless of how much you like them or how much they are like you. We saw that in the case of community/loyalty people tend to be biased towards those with whom they share a sense of collective identity. In the case of harm/care, people tend to be biased towards those for whom they feel empathy. If our moral universe consisted only of fairness, we would be outraged at the callous indifference people have for those outside their group and for those who fail to pull at their heartstrings. But like all human universals, these were adaptations for surviving in our ancestral environments. Early hominids spent most of their lives supported by their kin and menaced by their neighbors. It paid to be strongly biased towards individuals in their immediate community, with whom they already had strong emotional bonds. It was disadvantageous to feel sympathy for strangers in the next tribe. We no longer live in this environment, but our brains are still wired up as if we did.

Authority

In the summer of 2009, former United States President Bill Clinton traveled to Pyongyang to arrange for the release of two Asian-American journalists. They been captured and sentenced to hard labor in a concentration camp by the North Koreans for allegedly crossing their northern border with China some months earlier. The diminutive North Korean dictator Kim Jong-Il had wanted to meet in person with Mr. Clinton for a long time. The Dear Leader knew the prestige and respect such a meeting would bring him in the eyes of his pathetic brainwashed people. We've all seen the pot-bellied bastard waving to marching columns of stone-faced soldiers and little girls dancing with robotic precision on the official television channel. Image was his power. But Kim had recently lost a lot of weight in the wake of a debilitating stroke, and was reported to be suffering from terminal cancer as well. If there was ever a need for the insecure little potentate to save face and assuage his penis envy, this was it.

Bill Clinton probably had a few items on his wish list as well. Ever since his wife's defeat at the hands of Barack Obama in the Democratic primaries the previous year, the former president had taken flak for being selfish and out-of-touch with the American people. This was his chance to recapture some of the attention and respect he had enjoyed in the years before Monica Lewinsky, when he was the most powerful man on earth. In the end, a small humanitarian act was accomplished for the women, never mind that millions of desperate starving North Koreans still suffer and die in silence, never mind that the Dear Leader has his faltering fingers on the trigger of nuclear-tipped ballistic missiles aimed at Seoul, Tokyo, and perhaps Honolulu, never mind that his death will probably lead to a dynastic succession struggle full of chaos and bloodshed. What mattered were the images on television and the internet. On CNN, we saw two young Asian-American women tearfully reunited with their (white) husbands as the beaming elder statesman, Bill Clinton, looked on. On the North Korean state channel, there were images of a strangely rejuvenated Dear Leader proudly receiving apologies from the former President of the United States.

Respect for authority is a vestige of our animal lineage. Displays of dominance and submission are universal, not just in our species, but in all animals that reproduce sexually. It is a means of signaling who will get to mate and pass on his genes. It there were no sexual competition, and intercourse were random, strong and fit individuals would have little advantage over weak ones, and natural selection would be stymied. Authority is simply the extension of the sexual and territorial dominance common in the animal kingdom into the human realm, where it becomes formalized and codified. Because we are thinking apes who can delay gratification (sometimes indefinitely) and cloak our real motives beneath multiple layers of rationalization, the brute sexual and territorial natures of authority are not usually evident. But scratch the surface, and it's unmistakable.

Politicians and executives get the same boost of self-esteem from loyal underlings that they receive from adoring girlfriends. Contrary to popular belief, male sexual appetite has more to do with ego than with sex; rapists and sexual predators commit their crimes mostly for the sense of power it brings them, not because they're starved for sexual release. It's no wonder then that crooked politics and sexual indiscretion go hand in hand; the two are intimately linked. Politicians crave respect and authority as a proxy for sexual dominance. On the other hand, many women are sexually attracted to men who command respect and authority. But let's not get too cynical.

Sex and politics are both crucially important for social cohesion. If men did not compete for sexual attention, they would not pass on their genes; if men did not command respect and authority, there could be no society. One is necessary for the nurturing of children, the other for the nurturing of community.

In certain circles, authority trumps the other moral spheres. Authoritarian states like North Korea, Burma, and Iran use force and brainwashing techniques to intimidate their citizens into obedience. The strategy can be so effective that people will willingly betray their families for their leaders. North Koreans and Iranians are just as capable of fairness and empathy as anyone else, but they live in societies where those moral emotions are effectively squelched by cleverly pitting them against the equally innate propensity to respect authority.

Sanctity

Here are two more examples of moral dumbfounding from Haidt:

A family's pet dog is run over by a car. The family comes from an Asian country where dog meat is considered a delicacy, so they retrieve the carcass and cook it up for dinner. Anything wrong with this?

Julie and her brother John are backpacking across Europe on their summer vacation from school. One balmy night in the French countryside they decide that it might be fun and interesting if they tried making love. Julie was already taking birth-control pills, and John decides to use a condom, just to be safe. They both enjoy the sex but decide not to do it again. They keep the night their special secret, which makes them feel closer to each other. Is this okay?

Haidt presented these scenarios first to his students at the University of Virginia, then to undergraduates at dozens of other colleges and universities around the country, and finally to thousands of people of all ages in various countries around the world. Almost all respondents were unanimous in condemnation of incest, but there was some split on the first case. For example, undergraduates at the University of Pennsylvania who labeled themselves 'liberal' believed that eating the family dog was both a good source of nutrition, and an economical allocation of resources. When people who disapproved of the actions were asked why, many said they were simply convinced of a breach of propriety, but had a hard time articulating their rationale. Some standard weak replies included, 'a dog is a man's best friend', 'they might catch disease', and 'they might be sexually confused for life'. These arguments are easily shot down. But the most common responses reflected circular thinking: the actions were simply disgusting or immoral. But exactly *why* are they disgusting and immoral? Like the earlier example of the woman using a flag as a cleaning rag, these responses underscore two principles of morality. First, we base our initial responses on powerful gut instincts, and fumble to rationalize them afterwards. Second, some moral judgments are universal, while others are culturally variable.

Every culture has a set of issues that take on quasi-religious significance. In contemporary American society, these include gay marriage, teenage sexuality, abortion, vaccination, organic farming, school-prayer, and gun ownership, to name a few. Other societies may have different sets of touchy subjects that are classified as taboos or virtues. And within a given society, some issues that once pushed the buttons of purity and disgust in the past no longer do so (sex before marriage, single mothers), while others that did not, now do (spanking one's children, fur coats). As Steven Pinker puts it, 'there seems to be a Law of Conservation of Moralization, so that as old behaviors are taken out of the moralized column, new ones are added to it.' What is consistent in all cultures is that the moralization column always seems to have something in it. It appears that sanctity, purity, and taboo constitute a fifth moral sphere.

Haidt and the psychologist Paul Rozin have discovered that at the root of sanctity lies the emotion of *disgust*. Disgust is a human universal that evolved to protect us from infection. Substances that harbor disease-causing microorganisms such as feces and decaying flesh and the odors associated with them produce a natural revulsion characterized by an unmistakable facial expression and sometimes accompanied by a gag reflex. This emotional response was certainly adaptive for omnivorous apes that were constantly facing dining options that often came with life and death consequences. Those equipped with an instinctive alarm system set to go off at the sight or smell of potential disease-causing vectors had a selective advantage. Like so many other domains of the brain, the disgust module is deployed automatically and unconsciously, but it takes a while for the emotion to reach the cortex where it becomes a conscious feeling, complete with rationalizations and self-righteous excuses. And like other brain domains, once taken over by the rational system, it can be used for purposes other than for what it was initially selected.

The development of disgust starts around age two. Before this, nothing is disgusting; babies are likely to put anything into their mouths – including sterilized grasshoppers, imitation chocolate feces, and simulated rubber vomitus. This is followed by a critical period between two and four years of age when young children become increasingly finicky about what they will consume. It is almost as if some sort of neural pruning of indiscriminant dietary preferences is going on. Parents have a hard time, not keeping their kids away from bugs and feces, but getting them to try carrots and peas. After this phase, dietary habits harden and the set of disgusting things remains more or less constant over the rest of the lifespan. The list of what is considered taboo varies across cultures. In many parts of the world insects and grubs are perfectly acceptable, while eating pork or beef is beyond the pale. What is consistent is that these dietary habits are inculcated in young children by the example of their elders. Food taboos have little to do with preventing disease or promoting public health; they are almost entirely cultural or religious artifacts. But their violations can still provoke disgust in those who believe them.

Disgust is not only used as a response to forbidden foods, but can be extended to the other moral spheres as well. As our ancestors began to live in larger communities, there was an advantage to sharing common values and suppressing selfish desires. The emotion of disgust gave rise to its mirror opposite, sanctity/purity, and the two were then co-opted to help reinforce the moral emotions that people already possessed: fairness, empathy, community, and authority. Shared disgust (such as food taboos) and shared respect for common goals and good deeds acquired a religious aura that strengthened group bonds. Sanctity and purity are simply tools that our minds have fashioned out of the emotion of disgust and the magical thinking module to suppress selfishness and promote social cohesion. All political persuasions use the sphere of sanctity. Liberals deploy it to bolster fairness and empathy, while conservatives use it to buttress community and authority.

Let's return to the first two examples. It's safe to say that most Americans are disgusted and outraged at the prospect of eating the family dog, but people in Korea and Vietnam, where dogs are regularly consumed, might be equally offended at the notion of eating their pet pig. There is nothing intrinsically more dangerous or disgusting about dog meat than pig meat; both can cause diseases if improperly prepared. The difference is that in America, many families own dogs and children are taught to love them, not eat them. Because parents don't encourage their kids to eat dogs, the children develop a natural disgust at the prospect of eating dog meat, which they then pass on to their own children. The end result is that hundreds of millions of Americans who may have nothing else in common now share this collective distaste for dog meat. This shared trait is then recruited for the unrelated purpose of cultural cohesion. Communities, states, and societies are often molded by customs and food taboos, which may have had their roots in public health and hygiene, but eventually expanded into arbitrary cultural badges.

The second case concerns the more universal taboo of incest. There are good medical reasons for avoiding the practice. The confluence of recessive genes can result in offspring with terrible inborn disorders. Our ancestors undoubtedly noticed this correlation, ascribed it to some supernatural law, and frightened their children into avoiding the behavior at all costs. Unlike the practice of eating dog meat, genetic defects resulting from inbreeding have no racial or ethnic variation. Therefore, proscriptions against having sex with one's sibling or child cannot become a cultural badge designed to differentiate one tribe or nation from another; all cultures think it's wrong. But even so, rules against incest (or murder, or rape, or theft) work to strengthen the bonds within the community and serve as bulwarks against selfish sociopaths who might otherwise undermine the interests of the group by committing these acts at will.

Rules are easy to make, but notoriously difficult to enforce if they run counter to powerful selfish interests. One method of enforcement is to simply punish offenders with the goal of deterring them and others who may have similar intentions. Another is to reward those who play by the rules and keep on the lookout for cheaters. Both of these strategies rely on the reasoning, conscious brain. But, as we have seen time and again throughout this book, rationality is just the tip of a much larger mental iceberg. Strategies that work on the subconscious brain are much more effective. One way to uphold community values is to appeal to the emotions, especially disgust. A second is to engage the imagination, specifically its propensity for magical/religious thinking.

So to summarize, there are two possible functions of sanctity. Many things considered sacred or taboo are rooted in practices that have real physiological consequences such as infections, birth defects, and mental illness. But quite separate from that, all things sacred and taboo serve to bind communities together. Communities establish taboos by co-opting the natural instinct of disgust, and they sanctify things by co-opting the natural capacity for religiosity.

Politics

Each of the five moral spheres is an element in the periodic table of morality. Just as the atoms in the periodic table can combine to create complex chemical molecules, the atoms in the table of morality can combine to create complex social molecules. The elements can stand on their own, like the noble gases, or they can make exotic compounds, like lysergic acid diethylamide, but most of the time they hook up in highly predictable ways. In the chemistry of morality, the two most ubiquitous compounds are *autonomy* and *community*. Fairness and empathy combine to create autonomy. Loyalty, authority, and sanctity combine to create community.

Politics is the study of the reactions that come from the mixing and boiling of social molecules. Here are the fundamental principles. Liberals like to talk about nurture, education, the dignity of man, human rights, free expression, public safety, fairness, equality, diversity, and care. They criticize corporate greed, militarism, exploitation of the poor and the weak, and racial imbalances. Conservatives like to talk about human nature, character, virtue, self-discipline, hard work, free enterprise, responsibility, patriotism, heritage, and tradition. They rail against big government, unfair taxation, moral deviants, and the decay of family values. Liberals and western democracies in general cherish autonomy. Conservatives and non-western societies generally champion community.

Jonathan Haidt has discovered through online surveys that people who classify themselves as liberal tend to put greater weight on the moral spheres of fairness and harm, while downplaying the importance of community, authority, and sanctity. Those who call themselves conservative tend to place equal weight on all five spheres. Both sides believe with heartfelt conviction that they alone hold the moral high ground and that the other side 'simply doesn't get it'. Interestingly, these attitudes seem to be partly implicit and innate.

Why do liberals and conservatives consistently hold the views they do on such diverse and unrelated issues as taxation, the size of the military, gay rights, guns, affirmative action, and the environment? And why are they so emotional about them? The answer lies in both nature and nurture. The range of human politics comes from the interplay of individual personality and the cultural milieu. The 'big five' personality traits – neuroticism, extroversion, openness to new experiences, conscientiousness, and agreeableness – are now known to be highly heritable, meaning that they are closely linked to the expression of specific genes. They are the seeds from which the moral emotions arise. But just as seeds need soil, water, and sun to germinate, so too do individual personalities need communities, customs, and circumstances to develop.

Early in the twentieth century, the great trio of British experimental physicists, J.J. Thompson, Lord Ernest Rutherford, and Sir James Chadwick found that the chemical elements are not the smallest constituents of matter. They discovered the electron, the proton, and the neutron, respectively. Atoms are not dimensionless points in space but actually have internal structure. And in the 1960s, the American theoretical physicist Murray Gell-Mann discovered that these subatomic particles are themselves made up of even smaller stuff called *quarks*.

Another important concept is that physical reality cannot be completely described by the location and motion of matter alone. Electromagnetic waves, radioactivity, and gravity profoundly affect the behavior of atoms from the outside. Atoms are still the fundamental building blocks of chemistry, but physics can reduce their properties even further. This analogy works for politics as well. The moral emotions are still the fundamental building blocks of politics, but neuroscience and social science can reduce their properties even further.

Let's start with personality. The five basic personality traits are independent variables that become apparent in children by age two. They are shared by identical twins raised separately, but not by adopted and natural children raised within the same family. People can learn to modify or mitigate some of the more extreme elements of their personalities to adapt to their social environment, but, by and large, their characters are remarkably durable; people don't really change much. Personality is something we are born with because it is simply a manifestation of genes expressed in the brain to produce trends in thought and behavior.

Personalities, moral spheres, and personal political philosophies map quite nicely, though not perfectly, on top of one another. Those who are agreeable and open-minded also tend to be fairer and more empathetic, which, as we have seen, goes with autonomy and liberalism. Those who are conscientious and less open to new experiences tend towards loyalty, authority, and sanctity, which are associated with community and conservatism. Neuroticism, extroversion, and agreeableness can go either way. There are, of course, no such thing as liberal genes or conservative genes, Democratic genes or Republican genes; there are just genes that are translated into proteins which build brain circuits. But some of those circuits cause people to be more or less open-minded or extroverted, empathetic or loyal or domineering or religious, and those are the factors that help define a person's politics.

Politics does not come from human nature alone. External factors such as geography, history, and, more often than you might think, dumb luck are key players. In his celebrated book, Guns, Germs, and Steel, Jared Diamond makes a compelling argument that societies become advanced and aggressive or remain underdeveloped and vulnerable largely because of the agricultural resources available to them. People who lived on the great Eurasian landmass had access to a wide range of domesticable plants and big animals that they could harness to sustain large stratified communities. Those who lived in smaller less varied ecosystems such as the Australian Outback had to make do with less and consequently never developed advanced technology. One would therefore expect loyalty and authority, those community building moral spheres, to be somewhat more salient in large agrarian states rather than in small hunter-gatherer tribes. That was probably the case once upon a time, but things have become more complex.

The psychologist Richard Nisbett has done some intriguing studies comparing East Asians (Koreans, Japanese, and Chinese) and Westerners (Americans, Canadians, Western Europeans, and Australians) on tests of perception and cognition. The old stereotype is that 'Orientals' are tradition-bound, conservative, xenophobic, devoted to family, passive, effeminate, submissive to authority, ruthless to subordinates, and hard working, but lacking in creativity. Westerners are more open-minded, liberal, rebellious, aggressive, masculine, contemptuous of authority, generous to subordinates, and entrepreneurial. Like most stereotypes, there is at least some grain truth to this.

It appears that cultural characteristics can have robust effects down to the level of perception and attention. In one experiment (Masuda & Nisbett, 2001), Japanese and American subjects were shown identical scenes of fish swimming in a pond. When asked to describe the scene, the Americans tended to concentrate on the characteristics of the foreground: the big fish and what it was doing. The Japanese subjects concentrated more on the background: the smaller fish, the pondweed, the interaction of the fish with aquatic plants, and so on. It seems that Americans are concerned with the behavior of individual characters, while Japanese are more concerned about relationships.

These studies suggest that East Asians are more holistic in their perceptions and thoughts. Their attention is bound to the circumstances surrounding objects and events rather than to the objects and events themselves. This may explain the stereotypical Asian penchant for finding the middle way, compromise, non-confrontation, and resignation typified by feng shui, loose and flexible interpretation of legal contracts and religious doctrine, and the need to 'save face'. In fact, the Chinese language itself is much more context-based, rather than syntax-based like the Indo-European languages. Asian children learn verbs faster than they learn nouns, while the opposite holds true for Western children. Even the pictographic nature of Chinese writing reflects the emphasis on relationships and gist while the alphabetic writing of the West emphasizes precise definitions.

The origin of cultural differences is a highly contentious arena that goes back to the old nature versus nurture debate. Nisbett and many other social scientists are squarely in the top-down camp. While they may recognize the importance of genes as building blocks of biological and some psychological systems, they maintain that the elements of culture are purely arbitrary human constructs that are passed down and modified as societies evolve over time. One line of speculation is that contemporary East Asian societies reflect the characteristics of the ancient Chinese civilizations from which they sprang. Ancient Chinese culture was based on agriculture. The social roles and expectations of the people revolved around the strong cooperative effort required of rice farmers. As these people learned to live in tight cooperative social units over generations, their way of thinking, their language, and even their perceptions of the physical world took on a more context-dependent character. Although modern Asian culture has changed drastically in the last century as European Imperialism, communism, urbanization, and now American style capitalism have taken hold, fundamentally, East Asian society is still deeply influenced by cultural patterns originally set in ancient China.

Western society is largely derived from the Greco-Roman and Judeo-Christian traditions. Its two great wellsprings, the ancient Jews and the Classical Greeks, were, largely due to geography and environment, not primarily agriculture-based people. They were traders and merchants. The social roles and expectations of these peoples depended to a large extent on individual initiative and entrepreneurial resourcefulness. As these early 'Westerners' learned to live in highly competitive social environments over generations, their political philosophies, their language, and their perception of the physical world took on a more focused, individualistic, and object-dependent character.

There were times, such as the thousand years between the fall of the Western Roman Empire and the start of the Florentine Renaissance, when the characteristically aggressive mercantile spirit of Western Europe was suppressed by the crushing weight of religious superstition, economic backwardness, and catastrophic pandemics. Perhaps at such times, European culture and psychology took on a more Asian character. But fundamentally, and especially in the last five centuries, Western Civilization has reflected liberal cultural patterns first set by the Classical Greeks.

It is important to realize that politics is not race based. Like language and religion, the human capacity for political thought is genetic, but the particular language, religion, and politics a person acquires varies according to environment. Your mother tongue is determined by where you grow up. Your political beliefs are determined by where you reach social maturity. Chinese people think the way they do because that is the environment in which they develop, not because there is something intrinsically 'Chinese' about them. The intrinsic character of Chinese culture is the product of a particular history and geography, not something genetic in the people who happen to live there. Chinese immigrants who grow up in America or Europe will tend to think, talk, and behave like Westerners.

Modern Western culture is characterized by aggressive individualism because it is largely derived from the mercantile-based Greeks and Jews of antiquity (via the Roman Empire and Christianity). Eastern culture is characterized by passive collectivism because it is derived from the introspective philosophies of Hinduism, Buddhism, Taoism, and Confucianism. But it didn't have to be this way. The fierce Norsemen of Scandinavia became law-abiding conformists and even adopted socialism once they settled down to tend their farms. The Mongols rode out of their Asian heartland and conquered most of the known world with such bloodthirsty ferocity that no one would ever describe them as passive or effete. Genghis Khan left his genetic footprint on millions of people throughout Eurasia. Yet they too became passive once they were absorbed into the more collectivist ways of their Chinese subjects. Outer Mongolia even embraced communism for most of the twentieth century.

Liberals are happy that the United States has a New York City and a San Francisco. The two coasts exemplify all that is innovative, intellectual, and invigorating about America. But if the entire country were New York and San Francisco, it would fall apart. Liberals are too selfish to appreciate the commitment it takes to nurture large societies. Law and order, a strong military, family values, loyalty and obedience to family, community, and national authority, and the belief in God lie at the core of conservatism. Without them (and a continent full of natural and agricultural resources) there might never have been a large prosperous nation from which great liberal cities could emerge. Conservatism and community go hand in hand. I believe that they were the default position of all early societies.

The Taxonomy of Ideology

The bedrock values of autonomy and community are not sufficient to account for the differences between modern liberalism and conservatism. Liberals are as apt to speak about 'equality' as they are about self-expression and individual rights. Conservatives are just as preoccupied with 'freedom' as they are with duty, honor, and tradition. There is quite a bit of overlap between 'conservative Democrats' and 'moderate Republicans' both in rhetoric and in policy. Extremists from the left and right sometimes have more in common with each other than either do with their own centrists. To complicate matters further, there are two more players in the political spectrum that borrow key elements of the liberal and conservative philosophies without fully embracing either one. Let's try to make sense of the political landscape with some representative passages:

'To those peoples in the huts and villages across the globe struggling to break the bonds of misery, we pledge our best efforts to help them help themselves, for whatever period is required—not because the Communists may be doing it, not because we seek their votes, but because it is right. If a free society cannot help the many who are poor, it cannot save the few who are rich.'

John Fitzgerald Kennedy
Inaugural Address 1961

'The United States has no right to meddle in our domestic affairs. We do not speak English and we do not chew gum. We have a different tradition, a different culture, our own way of thinking. Our national character is different.

In the fighting in the Sierra Madera and in the fight with the mercenaries, many of our friends have fallen. They paid their final tribute. They did their part. We all have the same obligation to act with that spirit of duty, with that feeling of loyalty.'

Fidel Castro
Speech after the Bay of Pigs
Invasion 1961

'In the 1950's, Khrushchev predicted: we will bury you! But in the West today, we see a free world that has achieved a level of prosperity and well-being unprecedented in all human history. In the Communist world, we see failure, technological backwardness, declining standards of health, even want of the most basic kind—to little food. Even today, the Soviet Union still cannot feed itself. After these four decades, then, there stands before the entire world one great and inescapable conclusion: Freedom leads to prosperity. Freedom replaces the ancient hatreds among the nations with comity and peace. Freedom is the victor.'

Ronald Reagan
At the Berlin Wall 1987

'Government can never duplicate the variety and diversity of individual action. At any moment in time, by imposing uniform standards in housing, or nutrition, or clothing, government could undoubtedly improve the level of living of many individuals; by imposing uniform standards in schooling, road construction, or sanitation, central government could undoubtedly improve the level of performance in many local areas and perhaps even on the average of all communities. But in the process, government would replace progress by stagnation, it would substitute uniform mediocrity for the variety essential for that experimentation which can bring tomorrow's laggards above today's mean.'

Milton Friedman
<u>Capitalism and Freedom</u>

Liberals like John Kennedy have long appealed to fairness and empathy in an effort to champion equal rights. Liberal politicians have passed laws supporting progressive taxation, social welfare, public health care, protective tariffs, and government subsidies that force outright equality of outcome sometimes against popular resistance. Affirmative action is one particularly egregious example. This seems counterintuitive in light of the liberal philosophy of autonomy. Conservatives like Reagan have used the values of religion, tradition, and patriotism in their support for individual liberty. The Republican mantra of small government, low taxation, free markets, and the right to bear arms seems to undermine the ideals of a rigid stratified community.

The paradox of liberal and conservative ideology in modern American society can be understood if we break it down into two intersecting dimensions (Figure 16). On the vertical axis is the spectrum of social philosophy from community to autonomy. Recall that community consists of equal measures of the five moral spheres. Conservatives are strong supporters of community, so we can plot them near the bottom. As we progress up the axis, sanctity, authority, and loyalty fall away, leaving empathy and fairness behind. This is the domain of liberalism. But there is a second dimension we have yet to discuss.

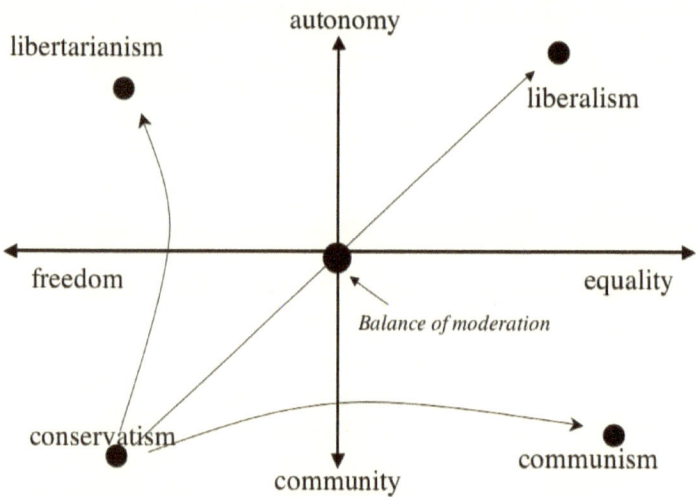

Figure 16: Political landscapes

Economic philosophy is concerned with how wealth should be distributed. It is quite distinct from social philosophy, which deals more with how communities should be organized. The spectrum of economic philosophy forms our second axis. At one extreme are those who believe that people should be free to amass as much wealth, comfort, and happiness as they can short of theft and coercion and should be at liberty to keep it or give it away as they see fit. At the other extreme are those who believe that each should be made to work to the best of their abilities and encouraged to provide everyone else with whatever they might need.

The addition of the economic freedom-equality axis to the social community-autonomy axis creates a new space for plotting political ideology. We are now ready to redefine the players. Conservatives are those who espouse community and economic freedom. Liberals believe in autonomy and economic equality. Those who champion autonomy and economic freedom are libertarians like Milton Friedman. Finally, those who support community and economic equality are communists like Fidel Castro. Picturing the political landscape this way is a bit artificial, but instructive in two ways. First, it helps us see the distinction between social and economic prescriptions for how people *ought* to live. Second, it allows us to imagine the natural histories of societies. I will address the first point later, but let's examine the historical aspect now.

I mentioned earlier that conservatism was probably the default political setting of the first human societies. This is because early humans – those sparse bands of nomadic foragers and hunters scattered throughout the Neolithic world – were steeped in the oral traditions passed down through countless generations of fathers and sons sitting around the campfire. They probably possessed all the moral spheres in roughly equal amounts, and they instinctively knew how to juggle them. But they had not yet mastered the art of inhibiting magical thinking, defying tribal authority, and suspending loyalty to the group. Nor had they worked out the kinks of creating a workable welfare state. Life in this less than idyllic state of nature was indeed poor, nasty, brutish, and short; the names of the games were every man (or family) for himself, dog-eat-dog, might makes right. But it is natural for men to have dreams and aspirations. Cavemen were no exceptions. As they sat around the campfire on cold dark nights looking up at the Milky Way, licking their wounds, and suffering the constant nagging hunger in their bellies, they imagined a better life where the spoils of victory would be more fairly distributed, personal opinions respected, and the slings and arrows of outrageous fortune would pale into insignificance in the context of a far greater common purpose.

There are three possible routes out of primal conservatism. They are the three utopias of *communism*, *libertarianism*, and *liberalism*. Over the last several centuries, all three trajectories have been tried with various degrees of success and failure. None of them are perfect, and each has their relative strengths and weaknesses. But one of them, liberalism, has had a better track record than any of the others. We will examine each of them and see why.

The Tyranny of Equality

The history of equality in modern Western philosophy starts with this famous passage from John Locke's <u>Essay Concerning Human Understanding</u>, written back in 1690:

> 'Let us then suppose the mind to be, as we say, white paper void of all characters, without any ideas. How comes it to be furnished? Whence comes it by that vast store which the busy and boundless fancy of man has painted on it with an almost endless variety? Whence has it all the materials of reason and knowledge? To this I answer, in one word, from EXPERIENCE.'

Locke's hypothesis of the human mind, which Steven Pinker calls 'the Theory of the Blank Slate', had an immense influence on political philosophy, psychology, and social policy for the next three hundred years. It can be argued that he did for social science what his esteemed colleague Sir Isaac Newton did for the natural sciences. The notion that all people start off with equal potential intelligence and ability is a highly attractive one to those who find themselves destitute, oppressed, and enslaved. 'We hold these truths to be self-evident, that all men are created equal; that they are endowed by their Creator with certain inalienable rights; that among these are life, liberty, and the pursuit of happiness', wrote Thomas Jefferson, a fervent admirer of Locke. Jefferson was motivated to write the Declaration of Independence in 1776 in response to what many American colonists felt was unjust treatment at the hands of their British masters. A century earlier, Locke was similarly inspired to write his Essay in response to what many Englishmen felt was unjust rule from their absolutist monarch, King James II.

The English people have long enjoyed a tradition of partnership or *social contract* between the ruler and the ruled, dating back to King John's granting of Magna Carta to the land barons in the fields of Runnymede in 1215. But that hadn't stopped some of his successors from flirting with absolute rule, most notably Charles I. When he dismissed parliament in 1640, the resulting popular revolt led by Oliver Cromwell culminated in a series of horrific civil wars we now know as the English Revolution. The royalists were soundly defeated at Marston Moor and Charles had his head chopped off. But Cromwell and his army of Puritanical zealots were just getting started. The fundamentalists expanded their holy war against the Anglicans, Scotch

Presbyterians, Irish Catholics, and even fellow Puritans deemed insufficiently pious. Meet the new boss; same as the old boss. After his death, a relieved population restored the monarchy by popular demand. But by the 1680's, James II threatened to become another Charles I. The specter of revolution loomed anew.

Locke was an astute enough student of his recent history to realize that while revolts kill their fathers, revolutions consume their children: a sobering lesson that would be repeated many more times in the coming centuries with increasingly horrendous consequences. Locke realized that the solution lay not in violence, but in reason. He envisaged the rule of law as a social contract negotiated between two willing and rational parties of equal potential ability and intelligence that agree to transfer power peacefully for the sake of strengthening the commonwealth. Injustices should be confronted with this argument: would an equal party agree to be treated in this way? Locke was encouraged by the relatively peaceful resolution of the latest absolutist crisis. In 1688, King James II was sent packing in the so-called Glorious Revolution.

As an armchair philosopher and defender of individual rights, John Locke was first rate. The only problem with his psychology is that he got it all wrong. As glorious as the revolution may have been, people are usually not all that peaceful, rational, or equal. To believe that they are so, and to base a model society on such presumptions, is to invite disaster. I have already discussed the violent and irrational nature of human behavior and its evolutionary roots. The same can be said for equality. Study after study has shown that much of the difference in temperament, personality, intelligence, and physical ability is inherited through genes. But people are not clones born with equipotent potential. If the justification for fair treatment is that people are naturally equal, the implication is that if people are not naturally equal, then discrimination is justified. But 'ought' does not follow from 'is'.

To be fair, Locke didn't actually think people were clones that could achieve equality of outcome in practice. He only believed that their mental capacities were roughly equal at birth because all minds start at zero: the *tabula rasa*, or blank slate. Thomas Jefferson didn't believe all men were really created equal either; he confided in numerous letters to his lifelong friend John Adams his observation that certain men were more or less industrious, thoughtful, or honest and that they seemed to inherit these traits from their parents. He paid lip service to equality in his Declaration because it was expedient to do so in the midst of a desperate war and because he believed in the *ideal* of equality. But ideals in the hands of great writers and leaders are potent forces of policy.

The French bourgeoisie were especially impressed by the success of the American Revolution, in which their seemingly invincible British archrival was finally humbled. They were also impressed that George Washington did not turn out to be an absolutist dictator in the mold of Oliver Cromwell or their own Louis XIV. These events seemed to vindicate the philosophy of Jean-Jacques Rousseau, the original hippie guru. Rousseau believed that human beings in the state of nature were basically 'noble savages' incapable of the institutional greed, corruption, and violence seen in modern society. 'Man was born free, and yet everywhere he is in chains', he wrote; the way to back to natural utopia is to throw off the shackles of authority and social convention. The idea of the Noble Savage stands in direct contrast with the conservative philosophy of the Englishman, Thomas Hobbes, who argued that human nature was inherently flawed, and that life in the state of nature was something to be abhorred. But if humans were basically good, Rousseau argued, the problem must lie in society. Reengineer society, and peace, love, and happiness will follow.

The French Revolution put Rousseau's countercultural theory to the test. Tens of thousands of young idealists from all over Europe poured into the streets of Paris lustily shouting liberty, equality, and fraternity. And thousands of them ended up on the guillotine upon orders of more radical minded revolutionaries. In terms of revolutions, it was more like the English than the American: the children were the ones consumed. It all ended with an egomaniacal dictator taking over and unleashing a war of continental proportions under the cynical pretense of spreading revolutionary ideals. Meet the new boss; same as the old boss. Romanticism may not have gone away, but Rousseau's dream of the Noble Savage was increasingly replaced by Hobbes' nightmare of the plain old savage.

In 1806, Napoleon's troops crushed the Prussian Army in the small university town of Jena. The spectacle of this world conqueror at the head of a vast revolutionary army captured the imagination of a young philosophy professor there named Georg Wilhelm Friedrich Hegel. Napoleon inspired Hegel to perfect his philosophy of idealism. In it, he tried to link everything from aesthetics and religion to epistemology, phenomenology, metaphysics, and natural history into a single unifying framework. At its center was the concept of 'geist' or organic spirit guiding history through the dynamic conflict of yin and yang – the Hegelian dialectic. For Hegel, history itself came 'alive' as an organic entity with conscious goals and desires. The role of the individual was reduced to an insignificant cog in a weird and vast machine. Hegel took the usual hocus-pocus of German philosophy to new levels.

Things could have stopped there, but when Hegel became essential reading for another impressionable young German academic, the left began to lose its way. Karl Marx came of age as Western Europe was undergoing its most wrenching period of industrialization. With his lifelong buddy and meal ticket, the aristocratic part-time socialist Friedrich Engels, he witnessed the plight of the disenfranchised working classes first hand as they toiled away in the dangerous and dehumanizing factories and sweatshops of Liverpool and Manchester. But instead of calling for organized labor reform, he believed that it was all a part of a gigantic pre-ordained Hegelian dialectic. Where Marx differed from his predecessor was in the role given to economic processes. For Hegel, politics and economics rest on top of the geist, the quasi-religious guiding spirit of history. In contrast, Marx was atheist. For him, religion (the opiate of the masses) and politics rest on top of an economic substructure. In effect, Marx turned Hegel upside down. But he agreed with Hegel that the fate of societies is predetermined in a natural progression that has no place for the personal feelings and desires of individuals. The exploitation of the working class is a necessary and inevitable step in the struggle towards the ultimate end of social history: universal communism.

Marx and Engels composed The Communist Manifesto just as Europe was convulsed by the revolutions of 1848. Workers and students in Paris, Berlin, Vienna, Prague, Rome, and many other cities erupted in mass demonstrations against repressive and reactionary regimes. They were crushed. But now, revolution had a new and far more radical voice. Forced into exile, Marx spent the rest of his life in Victorian England, where he wrote the communist bible, Das Kapital, and awaited coming of the worldwide revolution. He did not live to see the spectacular realization of his ideology. In 1917, Kaiser Wilhelm II sent an obscure Russian Marxist named Vladimir Lenin from Berlin to Saint Petersburg in a sealed railway car hoping he would infect the enemy with his subversive left-wing ideas. It worked, but the Russian Revolution came too late for the Germans to win the First World War. By then, Marx was dead and buried in London's idyllic Highgate Cemetery just opposite the right-wing social Darwinist, Herbert Spencer. Ironically, the nation he had adopted and hoped would lead the vanguard of the proletarian revolution was actually receding further and further from it. Communism's future lay to the east.

There are three major flaws with Hegelian idealism and the Marxism that emerged from it. The first is the denial of an innate human nature. The Hegelian/Marxist mind is simply a make-believe social construction. This is somewhat akin to Locke's Blank Slate, but much more literal. It implies that human minds and natures are infinitely malleable. The second stems from Rousseau's concept of the Noble Savage: the problems of the world come from imperfect society, not imperfectable humans. Reengineer society to the proper specifications and people will adapt to it. The third is the uniquely Hegelian notion of historical determinism in which individuals are just insignificant cogs in a quasi-organic process moving towards some predetermined goal.

Communism has an inherent appeal to outcasts who are too poor to own property, too disenfranchised to change the system, and too uneducated to distinguish fact from propaganda. These wretched masses made up the majority of the population in revolutionary Russia, China, Korea, Vietnam, and Cambodia. They were especially vulnerable to cynical rabble-rousers bent on using communist ideology to further their own selfish lust for power. Liberal educated idealists in these countries quickly realized how differently communism really worked compared with its promise, but for millions of them, the disillusionment came too late to save them from the gulags, re-education camps, and killing fields. Communism remained popular as long as there were formidable enemies to combat: exploitative factory bosses, racist social Darwinists, fascists, and Nazis. But as communist leaders became ever more despotic, and their societies became ever more inefficient, they became their own worst enemies.

Communism has failed, and the Berlin Wall has fallen, but at what price! Josef Stalin murdered as many as *twenty million* Russians through forced collectivization, torture, and execution, comparable to the number of Soviets killed by the Hitler's Nazis. Chairman Mao was responsible for the deaths of perhaps *twenty five million* Chinese in famines, deportations, and in re-education camps during the Cultural Revolution. Pol Pot massacred a third of his own population merely for living in cities, owning property, or being able to read. Two of the three worst mass murderers in human history were leaders of communist 'People's Republics' who paid lip service to equality. The fear of inequality and racism which first led genuinely humane liberal intellectuals like John Locke and Thomas Jefferson to champion equality had degenerated into the twisted ideology which allowed sociopathic monsters to torture and kill millions of innocent people.

Even today, there are some on the left who still cling to the theory of the Blank State. Fearing racism, sexism, and discrimination in general, they desperately maintain the hope that all people are really the same inside. They go so far as to deny the veracity of peer-reviewed studies that prove the existence of innate cognitive abilities in mathematics, social interaction, and language. Few of them are openly Marxist, but strip away the pretentious labels of multiculturalism, cultural relativism, deconstructivism, postmodernism, and political correctness, and you end up with the same nonsense. They believe that 'hard equality' or the imposition of equality of outcome is preferable to the unfairness imposed by racists and elitists. But is hard equality really more fair? Is it fair to punish someone because they happen to enjoy working harder, or because they are naturally more gifted? Is it fair to tax people more because they believe in saving for a rainy day or sacrificing for their children's future? Is it fair to legislate quotas on university admissions or job applications for the sake of ethnic diversity? Is it fair to make people feel that they should be someone they aren't and don't want to be because society would 'look more equal' that way? The answer is no. People are not equal in talent, temperament, or taste. To impose equality where there is none is as unfair as mistreating those who are less fortunate.

Postmodernists, poststructuralists, and deconstructivists are mostly pompous French bullshitters like Michel Foucault, Jean-Francois Lyotard, Jean Baudrillard, and Jacques Derrida who speak of reality as a social construction. It is true that perceived reality is a psychological construct, but it is not a social construct. By making a false leap from individual psychology to collective social phenomena, they have opened up a whole new system of errors. Postmodernists, like Marxists, believe that you can transform reality by reengineering the society above it, but this is all wrong. The only way to change perceived reality is to reengineer the psychology below it. And that can only be done by altering the biology at the bottom.

In order for the left to get back on track, they need a new conception of equality commensurate with their traditional focus on defending individual autonomy (which communism does not do) and maintaining economic fairness (which extreme socialism fails to do). The American political philosopher John Rawls offers a satisfying solution. He believes that in a society with a heterogeneous population of people with different innate abilities, interests, and philosophies, the fairest system of distribution is one that any given person would choose to live with, on condition that he make that choice under a 'veil of ignorance' of where his status would be in that society. In other words, let's say your chances of being born a beggar, a cripple, or a blind man are just as likely as you being born a rich, handsome ladies' man. If you were ignorant of your fate, what sort of society would you consider fair? Recall that in the second chapter, I discussed the concept of loss aversion bias, in which the sting of defeat is more intense than the joy of victory. If this holds true, I would expect most people to define a just society as a free market capitalist meritocracy (where the brightest and most motivated can rise to the top regardless of birthright) with a broad social safety net paid for by some degree of redistributive taxation (because it is less painful for a rich man to give some of his money away to help the needy than for a needy man to suffer without health and unemployment benefits). To quote Steven Pinker:

'Indeed, the existence of innate differences in ability makes Rawls's conception of social justice especially acute and eternally relevant. If we were blank slates, and if a society ever did eliminate discrimination, the poorest could be said to deserve their station because they must have chosen to do less with their standard-issue talents. But if people differ in talents, people might find themselves in poverty in a nonprejudiced society even if they applied themselves to the fullest. That is an injustice that a Rawlsian would argue ought to be rectified, and it would be overlooked if we didn't recognize that people differ in their abilities.'

'A nonblank slate means that a tradeoff between freedom and material equality is inherent to all political systems. The major political philosophies can be defined by how they deal with the tradeoff. The Social Darwinist right places no value on equality; the totalitarian left places no value on freedom. The Rawlsian left sacrifices some freedom for equality; the libertarian right sacrifices some equality for freedom. While reasonable people may disagree about the best tradeoff, it is unreasonable to pretend there is no tradeoff. And that in turn means that any discovery of innate differences among individuals is not forbidden knowledge to be suppressed but information that might help us decide on these tradeoffs in an intelligent and humane manner.' [Pinker, The Blank Slate pages 151-152]

Illusions of Freedom
In its broadest definition, *freedom* simply means an outcome that cannot be predicted. *Free will* is the ability to make a conscious choice between multiple possibilities. There's a fork in the road; I can go left or right. *Liberty*, in the political and economic sense, includes all of the above with the additional requirement that the choices are made with the knowledge of alternatives and consequences and without the pressure of time, stress, coercion, duress, or marked psychological limitations (such as post-traumatic stress, anxiety, or phobias). Liberty is usually exercised in the social and economic arena. Should I take the mortgage now or wait for interest rates to drop further? Responsibility is the flip side of liberty. In Western jurisprudence, people are generally held accountable for their actions when they are freely and willfully chosen with full knowledge of consequences. Crimes committed under such circumstances are fully punishable. One of the principal jobs of the criminal

defense attorney is to convince jurors of mitigating circumstances that would make their client look less responsible.

We make choices big and small every day. Some are important and life-altering such as whom to marry, where to live, which company to work for. Others are more mundane such as which movie to see, where to park, which size popcorn to buy. We take our freedom to choose very seriously because be believe that our choices and their consequences make us who we are. But how real is free will? Do freedom and liberty exist outside of our belief in them? If not, than how can we be responsible for any of our thoughts and actions? Let's dig deeper.

We can start with physics and metaphysics. The debate on whether or not the universe is deterministic goes at least as far back as the eighteenth century French astronomer Pierre-Simon Laplace. He postulated that if a demon (or God) were to have perfect knowledge of the position and momentum of every particle in the universe at a given instant in time, then he would in theory be able to apply basic mathematics to calculate the state of the universe at any other instant in the past or predict the state at any instant in the future. In other words, the future is totally determined by the past. If this were true, the reasoning goes, there could be no freedom, free will, or personal responsibility, since everything that ever happens was meant to happen in exactly the way that it does. The feeling of freedom we have is just another phenomenon that was determined at the moment of creation. There is nothing we can do about it: destiny is predetermined. There is a certain logic to this disturbing fatalism, and it is frustratingly difficult to disprove.

Fortunately, hard determinism was eventually disproven. In 1925, the 25 year-old German physicist Werner Heisenberg formulated the first mathematical description of quantum mechanics. It implied that an electron buzzing around the nucleus of an atom is located within a probabilistic cloud whose exact position cannot be pinpointed without interfering with its momentum. Conversely, its momentum cannot be precisely determined, even in theory, without scattering its location. Heisenberg had just discovered the *Uncertainty Principle*, which ranks along with Einstein's *Theories of Special and General Relativity* and Gödel's *Law of Unsolvablility* as Germany's three death blows against classical rationalism.

All particles, and indeed, all matter in the universe – including people, brains, neurons, neurotransmitters, genes, and so on – are subject to an intrinsic uncertainty built into their wave functions (discovered by Heisenberg's Austrian contemporary, Erwin Schrödinger). It is more marked the smaller and faster the particle: a photon might end up on the other side of the galaxy in an instant without violating the speed limit of light, for example. So we do not live in a deterministic universe as Laplace imagined, but rather a random one governed by the unpredictable laws of quantum theory. This again leaves no room for free will. How can randomness and chaos be compatible with deliberate choice? As David Hume famously put it, 'either the universe is determined, in which case there is no free will, or it is random, in which case there is no free will.'

But the behavior of large slow objects like planets, asteroids, and people is much more predictable. Their positions and momentum can be determined with *reasonable precision* by classical laws of probabilistic mechanics and thermodynamics, without having to invoke quantum physics. At the intermediate levels of size and speed, it is possible to leave out relativity and quantum weirdness, allowing for some degree of certainty.

That does not mean that we have to accept hard determinism either. The freedom to choose a particular action or thought is a function of brains, and brains are complex machines designed by natural selection. Although all machines, be they brains, bodies, or computers, are subject to physical laws (thermodynamics and quantum mechanics) at the most fundamental level, they are better explained by the laws of design (neuroscience, biology, computer logic). This is quite obvious to the biologist who would never attempt to use quantum physics to understand the behavior of a cell, or to the political scientist who would never imagine using cell biology to explain the behavior of social groups.

At the level of design, a type of freedom does emerge. It is the multiplicity of possibility. A machine can behave in unpredictable ways. The more complex the design, the more 'interesting' the possible outcome. There are only a finite number of interesting ways a thrown stone can fall. But a bacterial cell has rather more freedom of action. And a human being has even more still. The point is not what the final outcome actually turns out to be (there will always be one), but rather how many different interesting outcomes are possible given the starting conditions. Physics determines the final outcome, but design from selection determines the scope of possibility. So for our purposes, freedom is still alive. Now let's move on to free will.

Freedom emerges from design. But this freedom is not the same as 'free will'. Will means more than just possibility, it implies *choice*. The choice may or may not be conscious. In fact, we make unconscious choices all the time. Motor automatisms such as blinking are often unconscious choices. More to the point, the vast majority of the activity in your brain at this very moment is beyond the reach of conscious awareness. System one activity comes in the form of myriad parallel streams of neural pattern coursing through the re-entry circuits of the basal ganglia, thalamus, hypothalamus, amygdala, and other parts of the brain that make up the mind. As subconscious as all this activity is, it controls most of our behavior. This is not surprising given that consciousness is a recent development in animal evolution. All other species of life on earth do just fine with their unconscious choices.

It is an illusion that we are actually in control of most of our actions. The physiologist Benjamin Libet has done some very intriguing experiments measuring brain activity in subjects just prior to 'voluntary' behavior. The conscious intention to commit a voluntary act (flicking the wrist) occurs about 200 milliseconds prior to muscle action. But as much as 800 milliseconds *prior* to this (a full second prior to the act) there is measurable brain activity in the premotor and frontal cortex corresponding to the action. This has been called the *readiness potential* or RP. Libet believed that the RP is the subconscious signature of all voluntary activity. It originates in the subconscious and is accessed by consciousness after the decision has been made. If so, then we are never really in conscious control of our actions. There is no such thing as free will. But Libet went on to discover that RPs also preceded subsequently aborted actions. In other words, we can *consciously veto* subconsciously chosen actions. This has prompted Ramachandran to joke that although free will is an illusion, 'free won't' may be real!

To summarize, freedom of a kind does exist regardless of whatever degree of determinism or randomness rules the universe. This is because freedom of choice is predicated on the range of interesting possibilities allowed by design from selection. Furthermore, the size of the wave functions governing particles collapses at the scales of brains and people, allowing for some degree of certainty. But the choices and actions brought about by this freedom are largely unconscious: the end result of unmonitored brain activity. Consciousness, on the other hand, is a separate and, in some cases, separable process mapped onto all this underlying activity. Conscious will does not cause action; rather it continuously monitors and interprets the ongoing subconscious processes that cause our actions. And importantly, it has veto power to restrain otherwise automatic behavior. Our conscious interpreters believe they have free will, but they do not. Freedom is actually exercised by subconscious processes that enter conscious awareness a split second after the fact, giving us the illusion of free will. Natural selection has seen to it that the stream of consciousness closely tracks the subconscious streams of neural activity that actually cause our behavior. The tightness of this fit is the reason we usually feel so in control of ourselves. The psychologist Daniel Wegner has proposed a wonderful synthesis of these ideas:

'The experience of will is the way our minds portray their operations to us, then, not their actual operation...The real causal mechanism is the marvelously intricate web of causation that is the topic of scientific psychology... the real causal mechanisms underlying behavior are never present in consciousness. Rather, the engines of causation are unconscious mechanisms of mind...The unique human convenience of conscious thoughts that preview our actions gives us the privilege of feeling we willfully cause what we do. In fact, unconscious and inscrutable mechanisms create both conscious thought about action and create the action as well, and also produce the sense of will we experience by perceiving the thought as the cause of action. So, although our thoughts may have deep, important, and unconscious causal connections to our actions, the experience of conscious will arises from a process that interprets these connections, not from the connections themselves...' [Wegner, D.M. & Wheatley, T. (1999)'Apparent Mental Causation: sources of the experience of will' <u>American Psychologist</u>, 54, 480-492]

The Libertarian Fallacy

The modern formulation of libertarianism, the political doctrine based on freedom, comes to us from the writings of the great nineteenth century British political philosopher John Stuart Mill. Here is a sample from his famous essay <u>On Liberty</u>:

'...the sole end for which mankind are warranted, individually or collectively, in interfering with the liberty of action of any of their number is self-protection. That the only purpose for which power can be rightfully exercised over any member of a civilized community, against his will, is to prevent harm to others. His own good, either physical or moral, is not a sufficient warrant. He cannot rightfully be compelled to do or forbear because it will be better for him to do so, because it will make him happier, because, in the opinions of others, to do so would be wise or even right.'

'Over himself, over his own body and mind, the individual is sovereign.' 'Mankind are greater gainers by suffering each other to live as seems good to themselves than by compelling each to live as seems good to the rest.'

It is a convincing argument. Mill was a precocious child who was home schooled by his father James and his colleague Jeremy Bentham in the tradition of classical utilitarianism, the philosophy that the goal of society should be to maximize the happiness of the greatest number of its citizens. But the younger Mill eventually rejected this doctrine because it has offers no protection for minority rights:

> 'The "people" who exercise the power are not always the same people with those over whom it is exercised; and the "self-government" spoken of is not the government of each by himself, but of each by all the rest. The will of the people, moreover, practically means the will of the most numerous of the most active *part* of the people – the majority, or those who succeed in making themselves accepted as the majority; the people, consequently, *may* desire to oppress a part of their number, and precautions are as much needed against this as against any other abuse of power..."the tyranny of the majority" is now generally included among the evils against which society requires to be on its guard.'

Mill's conviction that the best defense of individual liberty lay in noninterference has resonated with libertarian thinkers ever since, among them the economist Friedrich Hayek, and the philosophers Isaiah Berlin, Karl Popper, and Robert Nozick, who wrote in his book, <u>Anarchy, State, and Utopia</u>:

> 'Our main conclusions about the state are that a minimal state, limited to the narrow functions of protection against force, theft, fraud, enforcement of contracts, and so on, is justified; that any more extensive state will violate persons' rights not to be forced to do certain things, and is unjustified; and that the minimal state is inspiring as well as right. Two noteworthy implications are that the state may not use its coercive apparatus for the purpose of getting some citizens to aid others, or in order to prohibit activities to people for their *own* good or protection.'

Mill is an admirable figure steeped in the great liberal tradition of British Empiricism dating back to John Locke. His true intellectual heir was the liberal humanist Bertrand Russell, not right wing Social Darwinists and proto-fascists like Herbert Spencer. But, as with Locke and the Blank Slate,

Mill's idea of libertarian minimalism was later incorporated into philosophies that grossly distorted the true vision of the original.

So what's wrong with a society based solely on autonomy and economic freedom? I think there are three main problems. First is the danger of Social Darwinism: the notion that 'might makes right', and that it is right for the strong to devour the weak. The second problem is that individuals left on their own tend to make irrational and often dangerous decisions. The third problem is that people are often happier when making choices within the context of community. Let's examine each of these three points.

The Social Darwinists and their more extreme cousins, the fascists, misapplied ideas of natural selection to social groups and cultural history to justify corporate greed, cutthroat capitalism, ethnic prejudice, and eventually genocide. They shared with the libertarians the belief that people are not equal in talent, taste, and temperament and that treating everyone equally is unfair. The points of departure were the notions that stronger is somehow better and that certain groups of people are superior to other groups. Mill never believed that; in fact, the main points of his philosophy were that the strong should defend the rights of the weak and that diversity of cultures, opinions, and personalities are what makes life worth living.

Many in the libertarian right defend their politics by invoking the myth of the Noble Savage. People are basically good, they argue, and leaving them free to do what comes naturally will bring out the best in them. Does it really? It is true that many private charities and philanthropic foundations thrive on individual freedom. But so do assault rifles, teenage pregnancy, and sub-prime mortgages. The truth is that people are neither all good nor all bad; they're a mix of both. The natural moral inclination towards generosity is offset by the equally natural inclination towards selfishness. If left unprotected, weak libertarian governments will inevitably fall to well-armed groups of thugs with their own agendas.

A good example of the conflict between freedom and generosity is health care reform. There are many on the right who oppose any form of government-sponsored health insurance on the grounds that they would lose access to expensive but potentially life saving treatments, such as new chemotherapeutic drugs. They argue that if they can afford to pay the premium on their private insurance, which would cover expensive treatments, why should they be forced to accept free public insurance, which does not? Life is sacred, they say, and allowing the government to ration health care is tantamount to letting them play God with the lives of innocent people. Former Republican Vice Presidential nominee Sarah Palin has likened President Obama's health plan proposal to 'death panels run by socialists.'

This argument is baloney for four reasons. First, health care is already rationed by the rising cost of private insurance, which makes it increasingly difficult for many middle and working class Americans to afford. Also, private insurance companies work hard to deny expensive tests, procedures, and pharmaceuticals to protect their own selfish financial interests often at the cost of the patients' interests. Second, the United States is mired in a trillion dollar deficit largely because of spiraling health care costs due to a combination of poor health habits such as smoking and junk food, defensive medicine, byzantine insurance company bureaucracy, too many emergency room visits by the uninsured, and the public misperception that the best medicine is the most expensive medicine. Third, many people believe denying any treatment is immoral. But this is actually selfish. The fact of the matter is that state-of-the-art medical care is a finite resource that cannot be given to everyone who needs it. It can be argued that it is even more immoral to leave 45 million uninsured Americans without access to any primary health care than it is to deny the most specialized or elective treatments to those who are insured.

The final reason concerns the value of life. Many agree with the Jewish proverb that he who saves one life saves the entire world; therefore, no cost should be spared to save any one life. This is just ridiculous. We put costs on human lives all the time. Life insurance companies and consumer product safety commissions routinely use standardized measures to calculate risks to life and limb when making guidelines on settlements and safety regulations. The philosopher Peter Singer has pointed out that health care economists have used the 'quality-adjusted life-year' or *QUALY* as a measure of the number of quality years a person in a certain state of health may expect to live. For example, people might come to a consensus that living ten years as a paraplegic is equivalent to five years as a healthy person. Advocates for the handicapped have angrily denounced the use of the QUALY as demeaning and discriminatory; they maintain that all human lives are of equal value. But Singer responds that if that were so, then there should be no benefit to curing paraplegia, a claim that no paraplegics would accept.

If all decision-making were up to free will, we would be masters of our fate. But conscious freedom is an illusion concocted by the interpreter after the subconscious parts of the brain have already decided its course. This leaves us with some major problems. We don't always do what we know is right. Take the case of obesity, a health care epidemic that costs the United States up to 150 billion dollars a year in additional costs (largely spent in the treatment of obesity-related disorders such as type II diabetes, heart disease, sleep apnea, and arthritis). Fat people know that they should watch their dietary intake and exercise regularly. But they fall victim to temptation and inertia. It is simply too difficult for system two to muster the conscious will power to inhibit system one from driving up to the takeout window at MacDonald's, getting the super-sized special discount meal, driving home, and plunking oneself in front of the remote controlled big screen TV for the rest of the night. If we allow things to run their course, more than half of all Americans will have obesity related diseases by the time they reach retirement, by which time social security may have run out. The free market won't save them. They need help.

The legal scholar Cass Sunstein and the economist Richard Thaler have come up with an idea that may work: *libertarian paternalism*. This philosophy, outlined in their recent book, <u>Nudge</u>, calls for the government to legislate measures designed not to coerce people to do what is good for them, but to frame their options in such a way that their rational brains have more of a chance of fending off their own irrational drives. Here are some examples that have already been put to good use: a certain percentage of your earnings will be automatically deducted from your paycheck and transferred to your retirement account unless you opt out of it; your organs will be donated in the unfortunate event of your untimely death unless you specifically check off against it; seat belts will automatically engage as you enter your car unless you manually disengage them. This can be applied to the case of obesity. Instead of punishing fat people by raising their insurance premiums or discriminating against them in the job market (or the dating scene), which already happens, why not tax carb-loaded junk foods and sugary sodas? We already do this with cigarettes. An ounce of prevention is worth a pound of cure. Why not put fresh fruits and salads *in front of* the usual hamburgers and fries in the school cafeteria display? Why not subsidize small organic farmers instead of huge corn-fed cattle farms that ship antibiotic and steroid laden meat to the fast food joints en masse? Libertarian paternalism is not dictatorship or a command economy, but a free economy with a human touch that helps people overcome their own built-in mental glitches.

My third and final point concerns the importance of community to freedom. Conservatives have long recognized that belonging to something bigger than oneself has its own special rewards. Aside from protection and support, community gives people a sense of duty and purpose that cannot be readily found in isolation. And studies have found that it promotes physical and psychological health as well. Recall the example from the second chapter about the young single attractive white man with the high paying job and beach-front apartment in Southern California? Chances are he is less likely to be happy than the middle aged married church going black woman with the working class job in rural Mississippi. This is because she has something greater than his money, house, looks, and even his freedom. She has the sense of belonging to a community. This is something that those who espouse the libertarian combination of autonomy and liberty should not overlook.

Go Your Own Way

The crisis facing humanity today is not the competition between the selfish and the cooperative aspects of our genes. That is a healthy competition that over hundreds of thousands of years has produced not just cultures and civilizations but even the conscious minds that can appreciate them. No, the real crisis is the conflict between the products of our genes and the products of our memes. Just like the toxoplasma-infected rat that unwittingly commits suicide, our species will likely wipe itself out sometime this century from catastrophic self-induced climate change, artificial intelligence, thermonuclear conflagration, genetically engineered pandemic, or some combination thereof. Unless we jettison our dependence on technology and go back to nature, we are doomed as a species. Human beings have become victims of their own success. They did not evolve to conserve resources; they evolved to be competitive and profligate. Humans were the first species in the history of life on earth to break free from the leash of natural selection and set the stage for their own downfall.

What then can be done to save us from ourselves? Probably not much, given the sorry track record of utopian movements over the last several centuries. But here are some hints for bringing the community of humanity together to face the global challenges facing us in the coming century.

Peter Singer has proposed the notion of the 'moral circle'. In prehistoric times, people applied the five moral spheres to the small bands and tribes in which they lived. All others were members of the out-group, to which empathy and fairness did not apply. As societies gradually evolved into cities, states, and nations, the moral circle expanded accordingly. Today, people routinely pledge allegiance to nation states, ethnicities, and religions comprising hundreds of millions of individuals. A liberal minority even expresses loyalty to the brotherhood of all humankind and to some of the more human-like species threatened with extinction. The logical conclusion would be for the moral circle to expand even further to encompass the entire spherical surface of this planet: the thin organic envelope we call the biosphere.

Jonathan Haidt calls for a more conservative solution in which liberals examine their own aversion to loyalty, authority, and sanctity. The left can learn much from the right. The conservative worldview is perhaps deeper and more in line with the minds of our ancestors who did not have the luxury of protection from a centralized government. If duty, respect, and reverence were universally applied to a fully enlarged moral circle that encompassed all humanity and the entire life-sustaining portion of our planet, then perhaps we could save ourselves as a species as well as we so often and so ingeniously save ourselves as individuals and small groups.

Steven Pinker has demolished the Theory of the Blank Slate with an inspired eloquence and common sense that is readily accessible to the common man. We would all be well served if we follow his teachings and accept that individual differences, whether rooted in nature or culture, do not justify unfairness and harm. All of us are born with a set of moral emotions that interact to create the motivation for human behavior. It is time we go beyond good and evil, nature versus nurture, and liberal versus conservative. Just as the nearly seven billion members of the motley crew of humanity all share one fragile ecosystem, the five spheres of the moral mind all share one limited consciousness. We should reject the old concepts of the blank slate and the noble savage and instead embrace the discoveries of behavioral genetics and evolutionary psychology with open minds and open hearts, for they are the true paths to enlightenment.

What we need is a society that respects the uniqueness of all of its citizens while providing a protective community that nurtures that uniqueness. As William James put it, 'without the individual impulse, the community stagnates; without the sympathy of the community, the impulse dies away.' Sociology is a messy science. There are no ideological utopias to be had in the real world. Hard freedom and hard equality simply do not exist; untold millions of human beings have perished in misguided efforts to reengineer society in their names. But we can do better if we aim lower. President Barack Obama often says, 'do not let the great become the enemy of the good.' Instead of equality of outcome, we should aim for fairness of opportunity. Instead of unfettered liberty, we should shoot for a variety of possibility. The British, with their usual understated approach, did it best. The most vehement critic of communism was an English socialist from the working class named George Orwell. The most implacable foe of the Nazis was an English conservative of aristocratic birth named Winston Churchill. The balance of moderation is an ideal to which all people should aspire.

Conclusion

Politics, religion, and decision making are three of the highest functions of the conscious mind. But, as we have seen in this book, they are largely beyond our control. Our illusion of being in command is based on the limited information that enters our consciousness. Only through scientific inquiry can we begin to uncover the tangled roots of thought lurking beneath it.

The first layer is the subconscious mind, first excavated by Sigmund Freud a century ago. Most of us believe that we simply are our conscious selves, occasionally biased by subconscious processes. The truth is the other way around. The human mind lies almost entirely within the realm of system one, and only a small part of it is influenced by conscious will. As counterintuitive as it seems, there is actually less to consciousness than meets the eye (and much much more to subconsciousness).

The next layer consists of the genes that encode proteins that build up the brain circuits that underlie our thought processes. Each of us inherits our full complement of genes from our parents at the moment of conception and keeps them for life. More than half of those genes are expressed in the brain throughout its development. The adult brain and the nature of its emergent personality are sculpted by genetic instructions encoded within each neuron. Environment and experience can regulate gene expression, but their effects are limited to the genes innately stamped into each embryo.

Beneath the deepest layer of genes lies the fertile soil of natural selection. The minds and brains we have today are the products of ancestral genes that built minds and brains best suited to survive and prosper in the Pleistocene savannahs of East Africa. Evolution is marvelously enterprising at creating genetic adaptations for better living. But it's a slow, tedious process. Our minds have created another adaptation for better living that works much faster: culture. The problem is that cultural evolution can outstrip the pace of genetic change, leaving us with outdated reactions.

Our behavior is largely controlled by subconscious mental processes resulting from the activity of brain circuits built up by genes inherited from ancestors living millions of years ago. The conscious mind is good at monitoring and interpreting subconscious mental processes, but doesn't actually drive most of our thoughts or actions. So are we just prisoners of our subconscious brains, developmental genes, and ancestral history? No, I believe we have more freedom than that.

The roots of thought extend from genes to proteins to neurons to neural circuits to brains to minds to cultures. Genes dominate at one extreme, while the memes hold sway at the other. Both are independent replicators. The conscious mind lies between the physical brain and human society, where it is buffeted by the winds of both genes and memes. We are not slaves of our genes, because our minds are largely shaped by parents, teachers, peers, and popular culture. Nor are we slaves of our memes, because our minds are also shaped by innate subconscious patterns of thought, hardwired neural circuits, and genes with unique histories. We are in between.

It has taken a massive multidisciplinary approach from many fields of science, including developmental genetics, evolutionary biology, developmental psychology, cognitive neuroscience, and evolutionary psychology, to unearth the roots of thought. All this remarkable research has revealed that the conscious mind is something very special, which has evolved just once in only one species of life on earth. Let's keep it going.